Get ahead!
The Prescribing Safety Assessment

Get ahead!

The Prescribing Safety Assessment

Muneeb Choudhry GP Director AT Medics, Undergraduate Tutor SGUL, GP Trainer, London, UK

Nicholas Fuggle Medical Registrar, Brighton, UK

Amar Iqbal Pharmacist, Heart Hospital, Birmingham, UK

Series Editor

Saran Shantikumar Academic Clinical Fellow in Public Health, University of Warwick, UK

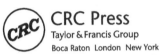

CRC Press
Taylor & Francis Group
Boca Raton London New York

CRC Press is an imprint of the
Taylor & Francis Group, an **informa** business

CRC Press
Taylor & Francis Group
6000 Broken Sound Parkway NW, Suite 300
Boca Raton, FL 33487-2742

© 2016 by Muneeb Choudhry, Nicholas Fuggle, and Amar Iqbal
CRC Press is an imprint of Taylor & Francis Group, an Informa business

No claim to original U.S. Government works

Printed and bound in Great Britain by Ashford Colour Press Ltd.
Version Date: 20160505

International Standard Book Number-13: 978-1-4987-1906-3 (Paperback)

This book contains information obtained from authentic and highly regarded sources. While all reasonable efforts have been made to publish reliable data and information, neither the author[s] nor the publisher can accept any legal responsibility or liability for any errors or omissions that may be made. The publishers wish to make clear that any views or opinions expressed in this book by individual editors, authors or contributors are personal to them and do not necessarily reflect the views/opinions of the publishers. The information or guidance contained in this book is intended for use by medical, scientific or health-care professionals and is provided strictly as a supplement to the medical or other professional's own judgement, their knowledge of the patient's medical history, relevant manufacturer's instructions and the appropriate best practice guidelines. Because of the rapid advances in medical science, any information or advice on dosages, procedures or diagnoses should be independently verified. The reader is strongly urged to consult the relevant national drug formulary and the drug companies' and device or material manufacturers' printed instructions, and their websites, before administering or utilizing any of the drugs, devices or materials mentioned in this book. This book does not indicate whether a particular treatment is appropriate or suitable for a particular individual. Ultimately it is the sole responsibility of the medical professional to make his or her own professional judgements, so as to advise and treat patients appropriately. The authors and publishers have also attempted to trace the copyright holders of all material reproduced in this publication and apologize to copyright holders if permission to publish in this form has not been obtained. If any copyright material has not been acknowledged please write and let us know so we may rectify in any future reprint.

**Visit the Taylor & Francis Web site at
http://www.taylorandfrancis.com**

**and the CRC Press Web site at
http://www.crcpress.com**

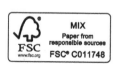

Contents

Foreword

I am pleased to have the opportunity to write a few words for this new book.

It is very clear that the need for publications which support clinicians in training such as medical students and pharmacists at the undergraduate and preregistration levels as well as beyond, to improve and support their professional practice, is essential. The content can also be of value to other healthcare professionals, for example nurse practitioners who are developing their clinical practice as prescribers.

I'm sure this book will prove invaluable to clinicians in training taking the new forms of preregistration exams in their chosen fields. The format is particularly useable because it is divided into eight clinical specialties of relevance to the newly qualified prescriber. These specialties are then cross populated into six prescribing safety areas: prescribing, prescription review, adverse drug reactions, calculations, interpreting data and how to communicate information effectively.

Throughout my career, I have sought to expand my knowledge and capability as the demands on newly qualified clinicians and indeed clinicians of greater experience have continued to grow. This book speeds up some of that learning and will improve clinical confidence.

I was one of the first pharmacists to train as a prescriber, initially as a supplementary prescriber, and my competency development was based on the limited resources that I had to identify through a personal trawl through documents, papers and assorted books. This book has collated some of that search into a readable and useable format to enhance the journey of learning and development.

I have found the book a delight to read, and I commend the authors on a very useful addition to the library of learning.

Ashok Soni OBE FFRPS FRPharmS
President (Royal Pharmaceutical Society)
LPN Pharmacy Chair (London)
Clinical Network Pharmacy Lead (NHS Lambeth CCG)

Preface

The prescribing of drugs or their antecedents goes back a long way: the journey from the apothecaries of old to the modern delivery of powerful and potentially harmful drugs has taken many hundreds, perhaps thousands, of years. Along the way medicine has developed, and mirrored scientific progress as it has done so.

So the 21st-century doctor has an armamentarium of medicines at her disposal, of which she will develop a knowledge through undergraduate and postgraduate training, and with the expectation that she will administer them safely and with efficacy. The learning that takes place is a complex journey and now is to be formally assessed under UK regulation, in its own right, in addition to the other examination processes regulated by the General Medical Council (GMC).

Drug prescription, having been formalized into a doctor-only process over the last century or so, has now been extended to other professions. So-called non-medical prescribing can be part of the professional development of many other disciplines: nurses, physiotherapists and podiatrists for example. Even pharmacists, whose relationship to medicines might be said to be closer than anyone's, can in the UK prescribe 'over the counter', pharmacist only and now 'prescription only' medicines (where they have done the appropriate training).

For doctors, the prescription of medicines has always been integral to clinical practice, and is assessed at an undergraduate level in final examinations. At the time of writing, medical schools have the option to include a Prescribing Safety Assessment (PSA) within their own assessments, or use the PSA to which this book is directed. Time will tell, but the PSA is likely to be the definitive prescribing assessment in the future. This direction of travel was set in train by *Tomorrow's Doctors*, a publication of the GMC.[*] Some of the thinking behind the establishment of the PSA by the UK Medical Schools Council and the Royal Pharmaceutical Society was well summarized by Rayburn in, appropriately enough, the *Student BMJ*.[†]

So the go-ahead young doctor will certainly get ahead by studying this book, which matches the structure of the PSA, examines the content

---

[*] GMC 2009. http://www.gmc-uk.org/Tomorrow_s_Doctors_1214.pdf_48905759.pdf

[†] Sayburn A. *Preparing to prescribe.* http://student.bmj.com/student/view-article.html?id=sbmj.h316

needed to be covered and offers support in examination technique. Having used this resource, or others, and passed the PSA, new doctors can claim to be safer in prescription, or at least to have demonstrated a good knowledge of drug safety. Given the estimated volume of drug-related iatrogenic disease, this is no small claim, and it is of particular relevance to the population health of the Western world, where multi-morbid elderly patients are at particular risk of this problem.[*]

Doctors when they graduate are taking on an awesome set of responsibilities, of which safe and efficacious prescribing is but one. They may certify death, be privy to very private information, excuse people from work, give professional witness to courts, perform procedures which invade bodily integrity, and see the raw emotion of the distressed patient. This list is not exhaustive, nor can it be, but it is interesting to note that we do not seek to assess the new doctor, by specific examination, in each of these areas of practice. We collate them together with other core knowledge and skills into 'finals'. It is a measure of the importance and risk of drug management that the PSA has been called into existence – and for which these three authors have produced such a comprehensive guide.

John Spicer MBBS FRCGP MA FHEA
Head of Primary Care Education and
Development, Health Education South London
GP, Croydon, UK

---

[*] Permpongkosol S. Iatrogenic disease in the elderly: risk factors, consequences, and prevention. *Clin Interv Aging.* 2011; 6: 77–82.

Acknowledgements

Muneeb Choudhry would like to thank his ever-supportive wife Asra, his son Ibrahim and twin girls Nabila and Saamiya for their patience, cheerful good humour and inspiration, without which this book would never have been possible.

Nicholas Fuggle would like to thank his wife Georgina and sons Jasper and Wilber for being eternal sources of inspiration, support and encouragement.

Amar Iqbal would like to extend a heartfelt and sincere appreciation to his family for having supported him throughout this endeavour. More importantly, he would like to praise God for having guided him throughout his career and for always being there when he has needed Him most.

About the Authors

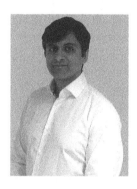

Muneeb Choudhry is a general practitioner (GP) and director of AT Medics. He qualified from St George's, University of London (SGUL), in 1998 and completed his GP training in 2003 in Croydon University Hospital Vocational Training Scheme. He travelled to remote and rural Australia after this as part of the Programme for Aboriginal Health. Following this, he completed a short service commission as a medical officer in the Royal Air Force. He then returned to the NHS to join AT Medics, London's leading Alternative Provider Medical Services (APMS) provider of primary care. He is a GP specialist trainer for the London Specialty School of General Practice and a Foundation Year 2 Clinical Supervisor, and he has also been a GP Hub tutor and Objective Structured Clinical Exam (OSCE) examiner for undergraduate medical students for SGUL. He is currently an appointed South London GP Appraiser and has also lectured at SGUL with an interest in prescribing. Additionally, he has developed practical expertise in minor surgery, joint injections, acupuncture, circumcisions, plastics and aesthetic procedures. Dr Choudhry is qualified in occupational medicine as well as in mediation. He holds additional posts as Learning Disability Lead in two Clinical Commissioning Groups (CCGs) in South London.

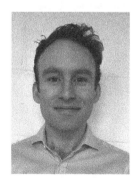

Nicholas Fuggle is a rheumatology registrar in Brighton and works with the Musculoskeletal Sciences group at St George's University of London. He qualified from Imperial College in 2009 and since then has completed his Core Medical Training in South London. He is a keen teacher and has held a post as honorary tutor at St George's where he lectured on clinical pharmacology. He has a research interest in the aetiology of inflammatory arthritis and has presented nationally and internationally. His prizes include The St Mary's Association Prize, The Association of Clinical Pathologists Incentives Prize and Scholar of the World Congress of Dermatology.

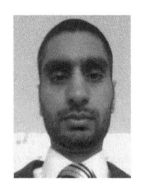

Amar Iqbal is currently deputy chief pharmacist at Birmingham Women's Hospital, Birmingham, UK. He qualified with first class honours from Aston University, Birmingham, UK, in 2007 and completed his training year with Alliance-Boots, where he went on to become a store manager at the first ever hospital outpatient pharmacy collaboration in the United Kingdom. He switched to the National Health Service (NHS) in 2010, where he gained broad experience in dermatology, adult medical wards, surgical wards, emergency admissions, neurorehabilitation wards and medicines information amongst others whilst at Sandwell and West Birmingham Hospitals NHS Trust. Amar also gained experience in ophthalmology at Birmingham and Midland Eye Clinic.

Amar joined Heart of England NHS Foundation Trust (HEFT) in 2012 as a women's and children's health pharmacist, where he attended to a level 3 neonatal intensive care unit (NICU), general paediatric wards (including high dependency unit), surgical day cases, and obstetrics and gynaecology. He also provided support to the paediatric emergency department, maternity wards and some outpatient clinic areas. He also worked closely on the training and education of doctors and nurses in the NHS. This included working on an in-house prescribing training module (VITAL). During his time with HEFT, Amar was seconded to a teacher–practitioner role, where he worked with students from Aston University on patient-focused learning and assessment within the hospital and university setting. Locally, Amar has created an introductory prescribing module for West Midlands Deanery as part of the SCRIPT eLearning initiative for specialist paediatric trainees.

After leaving HEFT in 2015, Amar was director of a professional consultancy firm and also worked as a locum pharmacist which brought him back to adult medical and surgical specialities.

Amar is a keen advocate of the Royal Pharmaceutical Society and for the past five years has had a dedicated role as pre-registration and student development lead at Birmingham and Solihull Local Practice Forum. Amar has also worked for both professional (RPSGB) and regulatory bodies (GPhC) for pharmacy whilst contributing to local and national initiatives and guidelines.

Introduction

Prescribing forms a major part of the workload of doctors in their foundation years; it is a complex task which requires careful attention and due diligence. It requires you as a prescriber to be familiar with the use, side effect profile and risks and benefits of various medications.

The prescribing process is full of dangers, and literature shows prescribing errors to be part of this. A recent study (EQUIP) found that 9% of hospital prescriptions contained an error. With this in mind, the General Medical Council initially (in 2013) piloted and has now (in 2014) put into place a national prescribing safety assessment that allows you to demonstrate your core prescribing competencies. The assessment is a joint collaboration between the British Pharmacological Society and the Medical Schools Council that aims to allow for safe and effective prescribing for the betterment of patient health.

Core prescribing competencies include, among others:

- Writing new prescriptions
- Reviewing existing prescriptions
- Amending prescriptions to suit individual patient profiles
- Identifying adverse drug reactions
- Identifying and avoiding medication errors
- Calculating doses

Medical schools still have the choice of compiling their own equivalent exam, which has to be of the same or higher level of difficulty, to assess the same competencies (as judged by an external panel). This may be in an electronic or written format which will provide a small degree of variation in technique required to complete the assessment. This is due to the fact that you may be clicking with a mouse on boxes or opening the Electronic British National Formulary (eBNF) on a computer-based exam, as opposed to filling in boxes with a pencil and physically turning the pages of the BNF hard copy, in the written format.

Using the BNF and eBNF as much as possible during the revision period is extremely helpful, as the more familiar you are with the formats and tools embedded within it, the less time you will spend searching during the exam.

STRUCTURE OF PSA

The PSA is marked as either 'pass' or 'fail'. It assesses the skills, judgement and supporting knowledge that relate to medical prescribing of all final-year medical students. It consists of eight different question types, each of which is defined under seven subsets of clinical activity:

Question type	Clinical activity subset
Prescribing	
Prescription Review	Medicine
Planning Management	Surgery
Communicating Information	Elderly Care
Calculation Skills	Paediatrics
	Psychiatry
Adverse Drug Reactions	Obstetrics and Gynaecology
Drug Monitoring	General Practice
Data Interpretation	

Each question can be classified in two different ways – either by question type or by the clinical specialty being tested.

LAYOUT OF PSA

Section 1	8 items	Questions in each section
Prescribing	(10 marks each) 80 marks	can relate to any of the
Section 2	8 items	following seven subsets of
Prescription Review	(4 marks each) 32 marks	clinical activity:
Section 3	8 items	Medicine
Planning Management	(2 marks each) 16 marks	Surgery
Section 4	6 items	Elderly Care
Communicating Information	(2 marks each) 12 marks	Paediatrics
		Psychiatry
Section 5	8 items	Obstetrics and Gynaecology
Calculation Skills	(2 marks each) 16 marks	General Practice
Section 6	8 items	
Adverse Drug Reactions	(2 marks each) 16 marks	
Section 7	8 items	
Drug Monitoring	(2 marks each) 16 marks	
Section 8	6 items	
Data Interpretation	(2 marks each) 12 marks	
TOTAL	**TOTAL**	
8 sections	60 items/200 marks	

- You will have **2 hours** (120 minutes) in which to do the PSA.
- The 'pass' mark will vary depending on the difficulty of the questions. The information pertaining to the 'pass' mark will be included when you log into the PSA examination interface.

QUESTION STRUCTURE AND LAYOUT

Below is a brief summary of the layout of the question types you may encounter in your assessment. In the pages following this is an explanation of each section of the assessment with a list of potential common prescribing issues you may be examined on.

Section	Question type
Prescribing	Write a prescription for ONE drug that will help to [*treat/alleviate/prevent*] [*symptom or problem*]. *(Use the hospital [name of chart type]/general practice prescription chart provided)*
Prescription Review	Select the [*ONE/TWO/THREE prescription/prescriptions*] that [*is/are*] [*most likely* to be] [a cause of/contains a serious dosing error/interact/contraindicated etc.]. *(Mark [it/them] with a tick in column [A/B])*
Planning Management	Select the *most appropriate* management option at this stage. *(Mark it with a tick)*
Communicating Information	Select the *most appropriate* information option that should be provided for the [*patient/mother/staff nurse/GP*]. *(Mark it with a tick)*
Calculation Skills	What is the [*total amount/volume/duration/total dose etc.*] that the patient [*should be given etc.*] …? *(Write your answer in the box below)*
Adverse Drug Reactions	**Type A** – 'Select the adverse effect that is *most likely* to be caused by this treatment. *(Mark it with a tick)*' **Type B** – 'Select the prescription that is *most likely* to be contributing to [*describe the clinical problem here*]. *(Mark it with a tick)*' **Type C** – 'Select the prescription that is *most likely* to interact with [*the drug specified in the stem*] to [*describe the clinical problem here*]. *(Mark it with a tick)*' **Type D** – 'Select the *most appropriate* option for the management of this adverse drug reaction. *(Mark it with a tick)*'
Drug Monitoring	Select the *most appropriate* monitoring option to assess the [*beneficial/adverse*] effects of this treatment. *(Mark it with a tick)*
Data Interpretation	Select the *most appropriate* decision option with regard to [*the prescription/the treatment of*] based on these data. *(Mark it with a tick)*

CLINICAL SUBSETS EXPLAINED

Clinical subset	Question type
Medicine	This subset will cover the following areas: **Admissions Cardiovascular Gastroenterology Neurology Rheumatology** Common medical emergencies can also be covered here too.
Surgery	This subset will cover pre-operative and post-operative surgery in areas such as: **Colorectal General surgery Trauma and orthopaedics**
Elderly Care	This subset will look at elderly patients and problems such as: **Dementia Incontinence Poly-pharmacy Stroke**
Paediatrics	This subset will look at neonates and children up to the age of 16 years.
Psychiatry	This subset will cover common psychiatric problems such as: **Anxiety Behavioural Depression Psychotic** **disturbances symptoms**
Obstetrics and Gynaecology	This subset will look at perinatal and antenatal care in women. It will also look at those women using contraception, and common gynaecological problems such as: **Bleeding Infections Menstrual cycle Sexual health** **disorders disorders issues**
General Practice	This subset will cover common problems encountered in primary care. This will cover areas such as: **Dermatology ENT issues Immunizations Ophthalmology**

HIGH-RISK DRUGS

You will be expected to know about high-risk prescribing drugs as per National Patient Safety Agency (NPSA) advice. High-risk drugs are those which are known to have caused, or have the potential to cause, severe harm and/or death. The assessment will expect you to look at least one of the following agents listed below.

Agent(s)	What you may be expected to know about
Antibiotics	• Different types of antibiotics (including structural similarities – e.g. penicillins vs carbapenems vs cefalosporins – and differences) • Likely effects of missed/omitted doses • Drugs that require therapeutic monitoring • Gentamicin double-checking prompt sheet (for neonates) • Common and/or serious interactions between antibiotics and drugs
Anti-coagulants	• Uses of older and newer anti-coagulants • Likely effects of missed/omitted doses • Side effect profile and monitoring/adjustments required • Warfarin and interactions with other drugs/food and drink • How to deal with excessive anti-coagulation • Heparin products (e.g. strengths) and their uses (including as flushes) • Use of multiple anti-coagulation agents and associated risk/benefit
Insulin	• Different types of insulin (including their profiles) • Likely effects of missed/omitted doses • Safely prescribing insulin products (including sliding scale insulin) • Dosing and monitoring of insulin preparations (including harm of long-term hyperglycaemia that is not adequately managed) • Managing hypoglycaemia
Infusion fluids	• Different types of infusion fluids, when they are used and why • Hypertonic versus hypotonic versus isotonic fluids (e.g. sodium chloride) • Calculating fluid replacement • Prescribing of infusion fluids • Appropriate electrolyte replacement therapy
Opioid analgesics	• WHO analgesic ladder • How to prescribe controlled drugs and PCA drugs • Dose conversions between drugs • Opioid naïve patients • Palliative care prescribing • Side effect and haemodynamic profile • Drug–drug interactions and increased risk of side effects (e.g. respiratory depression)

You will **not be expected to know about anaesthetic, chemotherapy and antipsychotic agents** as these are normally initiated by a specialist.

SECTION 1: PRESCRIBING

- Eight questions (10 marks each).
- Requires you to prescribe a medication in response to a given clinical scenario.
- You will need to review the clinical situation and any additional information to decide upon:
  - The most appropriate medication to prescribe
  - The most appropriate dose, route and frequency for this medication
- You will be assessed on your ability to write a safe, effective and legal prescription.
- The question will outline a clinical scenario and ask you to write a prescription on an electronic prescription chart. This may be as a regular medication, as a STAT dose, as a PRN dose or as a fluid chart prescription.
- Common conditions or areas that you will need to be aware of (N.B. this is not an exhaustive list) include:

Acute conditions	Acute asthma, acute MI, anaphylaxis, VTE prophylaxis, infections
Chronic conditions	COPD, depression, diabetes, heart failure, hypertension

- You will also be expected to distinguish between **important symptoms** such as pain, breathlessness or headache.
- You will be expected to make an appropriate choice of medication based on
  - The available products
  - The different types of formulations
  - The available access points and routes
  - The dose frequency
- One key tip is that you must utilize the approved name (i.e. the drug name) when prescribing a drug. This is sometimes termed 'generic prescribing' and the drug name is written as a 'generic name', for example prescribing as 'paracetamol' as opposed to 'Panadol®'.

- Only use brand names where clinically necessary:

Reason for using the brand (proprietary) name when prescribing	Example(s)
When there is a significant difference in bioavailability between formulations (i.e. where the fraction of dose available for therapeutic effect will differ from preparation to preparation).	Beclamethasone inhalers (e.g. QVAR®) Carbamazepine (e.g. Tegretol®) Ciclosporin (e.g. Neoral®)
For some narrow therapeutic index drugs where the difference between therapeutic and toxic levels is small.	Lithium (e.g. Priadel®) Theophylline (e.g. Uniphyllin®)
Where you cannot interchange between preparations due to:	
1. The type of formulation (e.g. modified released product where the dosing frequency is different, or insulin products)	Adalat® LA vs Adalat® Retard
2. Availability of various products of a similar type	Betnovate® vs Betnovate-RD®
3. Subtle difference in formulation (e.g. concentrated vs diluted creams)	Humalog® vs Humalog® Mix25 Microgynon®30 vs Ovranette®
Where a product contains more than one ingredient or comes in variable strengths (of differing brands) and a brand name will help to easily identify it.	Gaviscon® vs Peptac® Creon® 10,000 vs Creon® 25,000 Movicol® vs Movicol® Plain

- The table below is not an exhaustive list of common drugs or classes of drugs that you may need to prescribe by the brand name.

Common drugs where you will need to specify the brand name when prescribing

Approved name/ class of drug	Common brands	Approved name/ class of drug	Common brands
Aminophylline	Phyllocontin Continus®, Phyllocontin Continus Forte® etc.	Insulins	Humalog®, Humulin®, NovoRapid®, Levemir®, Lantus® etc.
Antacids	Gaviscon®, Peptac®, Maalox® etc.	Lithium	Camcolit®, Liskonum®, Priadel® etc.
Azathioprine	Azamune®, Imuran® etc.	Mesalazine	Asacol®, Pentasa® etc.
Beclomethasone (inhaler devices)	QVAR®, Clenil® Modulite	Methylphenidate	Equasym® XL, Medikinet® XL, Ritalin®, Concerta® XL etc.
Carbamazepine	Carbagen® SR, Tegretol®, Tegretol Retard® etc.	Mycophenolate	Arzip®, CellCept® etc.
Ciclosporin	Neoral®, Sandimmune®	Nifedipine	Adalat®, Adalat® LA, Adalat Retard®, Coracten® XL, Fortipine®, Nifedipress®, Tensipine® etc.
Compound haemorrhoid preparations	Anusol®, Anusol HC®, Proctosedyl®, Scheriproct® etc.	Pancreatin	Creon®, Creon® Micro, Pancrex®, Pancrease® HL etc.
Diltiazem	Adizem® SR, Adizem® XL, Angitil® SR, Angitil® XL, Dilzem® SR, Slozem®, Tildiem® LA, Tildiem Retard®, Viazem® etc.	Skin or eye preparations	Dermol® 500 lotion, Diprobase® cream, Hydromol® cream, Locotern-Vioform®, Cosopt® etc.
Estradiol (and other hormonal or contraceptive patches)	Estradot®, Evorel®, FemSeven® etc.	Tacrolimus	Adoport®, Capexion®, Modigraf®, Prograf®, Tacni®, Vivadex®
Fentanyl patches	Durogesic® D-Trans, Tilofyl® etc.	Theophylline	Nuelin® SA, Slo-Phyllin®, Uniphyllin Continus®

- Do not use abbreviations for drug names or doses. Some common examples of this are:
  - Do not prescribe AZT for azathioprine.
  - Do not prescribe FeSO$_4$ for ferrous sulfate.
  - Do not prescribe MTX for methotrexate.
  - Do not prescribe NaCl for sodium chloride 0.9%.
  - For insulin products, write the units in full (e.g. 2 units TDS).
  - For microgram and nanogram doses, please write the units in full (**do not** write mcg or μg or ng).

- Provide any other relevant instructions or details (e.g. special administration instructions).
- Sign and date your prescription, and also write any dose timings.
- Some drugs have doses which are not once daily; be familiar with these:

Drug(s)	Usual dosing schedule
Bisphosphonates	Alendronic acid (alendronate) – 70 mg once weekly Risendronic acid (risedronate) – 35 mg once weekly
Buprenorphine	Patches are usually changed once weekly
Fentanyl	Patches are changed every 72 hours (i.e. every 3rd day)
Hyoscine	
Hydroxocobalamin	1 mg three times a week for 2 weeks, then 1 mg every 2 or 3 months (depending on type of anaemia)
Gentamicin	Given every 36 hours in premature neonates (as opposed to every 24 hours)
Methotrexate	Given once weekly

- Remember to always consider any allergy details (where provided).
- With respect to penicillin allergies, you will need to look out for the following:
  - **Is it a true allergy (anaphylaxis/hypersensitivity vs minor sensitivities such as rash confined to a small area or delayed rash presentation)?** Where a risk of immediate hypersensitivity is suspected, do not prescribe a penicillin or related drug.
  - **Does the patient have an atopic history (e.g. asthma, eczema and hay fever)?** These patients are at higher risk of anaphylactic reactions and should receive a penicillin or related drug with caution.
  - **Penicillin-based drugs and related drugs include:**
    - Carbapenems (imipenem, meropenem etc.)
    - Cefalosporins (cefalexin, ceftazidime, ceftriaxone etc.) due to cross-reactivity (1)
    - Monobactams (aztreonam – although this is less of a culprit and can be used cautiously)
    - Combination products such as 'co-amoxiclav' (also known as 'Augmentin®') should also be avoided

The mark breakdown currently for the prescribing section is as follows:

Drug choice	4 marks
Dose/route/frequency	4 marks
Timing	1 mark
Signature	1 mark

Where 4 marks are allocated, there is a reducing scale; in essence, you can lose marks based on a sub-optimal response. Reasons for a sub-optimal response include:

- Lack of clinical effectiveness
- Expensive drug choice
- Lack of availability of a drug in a given clinical setting
- Issues with tolerability and/or adherence (e.g. infant unable to swallow tablets)
- Propensity for a drug interaction

SECTION 2: PRESCRIPTION REVIEW

- Eight questions (4 marks each).
- Requires you to **analyse** a list of five or more currently prescribed medications.
- It is assumed that you will have some **knowledge** of **common effects**, **adverse reactions** and **common interactions**. *You will need to decide which medication(s) is/are inappropriate, unsafe or unlikely to be effective based on the patient details provided.*
- You will be assessed on your ability to **identify unsafe prescriptions** (based on dose, route or actual drug) from a list of medications. This may be an extract from a drug chart, a referral letter or other healthcare documentation. You will need to **assess** this list of medications based on a given **clinical problem**, which may include:
  - Hepatic or renal impairment
  - Loss of anti-coagulation control
  - Headache or other clinically important symptoms
- **Problems that you may need to identify will include:**
  - Common or serious drug interactions
  - Obvious or serious dosing errors
  - Sub-optimal prescribing

Common or serious drug interactions	Obvious or serious dosing errors	Sub-optimal prescribing
• Amiodarone with warfarin	• Analgesic dosing	• Steroids given in the evening
• Clarithromycin with simvastatin	• Dosing of narrow therapeutic index drugs (e.g. theophylline, digoxin etc.)	• Loop diuretics or drugs with a stimulant effect given late in the day (after 2 p.m. or 4 p.m. respectively)
• Verapamil with beta-blockers	• Exceeding adult maximum dose for a drug	• Sub-therapeutic doses (e.g. low dose of antibiotic)
• Diltiazem and verapamil with digoxin	• Dose frequency incorrect (e.g. once-daily preparation given twice daily)	• Standard preparation prescribed instead of M/R or vice versa
• Food with phenytoin	• Dose given as a single daily dose when it should be a divided dose • Dose given as a daily dose when it should be a weekly dose	

SECTION 3: PLANNING MANAGEMENT

- Eight questions (2 marks each).
- Requires you to utilize reason and judgement to decide which combination of therapies is appropriate to manage a particular clinical patient scenario.
- You will be given a clinical scenario and asked to detail the **most suitable** *or* **best therapeutic strategy** that should form part of the **initial management** of the given patient.
- You will be expected to select between suitable options which may include a drug, a fluid or other medical strategies (such as a TENS unit for pain relief, cognitive behavioural therapy and physiotherapy). The option you choose would be the one which is of most benefit compared to the others.
- Remember to consider patient signs and symptoms, and any investigations which may help guide you to a suitable treatment option.
- The treatment options may be preventative, curative, symptomatic or palliative.
- **Scenarios can include management of clinical toxicological emergencies:**
  - Acute overdoses
  - Alcohol or other types of poisoning
  - Acid–base disturbances
  - Fluid–electrolyte imbalances
- Although the diagnosis or differential diagnosis will be clear from the given information, you will not need to deduce what it is. This is to reflect real-life scenarios where planning management is important even when the underlying diagnosis is uncertain.

SECTION 4: COMMUNICATING INFORMATION

- Six questions (2 marks each).
- You will be given a brief scenario in which a patient is due to start a new treatment or needs advice about existing treatment.
- Requires you to identify the most appropriate information that you need to provide the patient in order to either:
  - Allow them to choose whether to take the medicine or not
  - Enhance the safety and effectiveness of a medication
- You will have a list of five options to choose from; four will be plausible distractors.

SECTION 5: CALCULATION SKILLS

- Eight questions (2 marks each).
- You will need to accurately calculate and correctly record (with units) dosing based on numerical information.
- **The scenarios may include:**
  - **Dose of a drug** based on:
    - Age
    - Weight
    - Body surface area
  - **Rate** of administration of a drug or fluid
  - **Quantity** of tablets required to give a set dose
  - **Dose adjustments** based on clinical parameters or bioavailability
  - **Drug and fluid dilutions** for administration in an infusion pump
  - Your ability to **utilize** and/or **convert** between **units or concentrations**

SECTION 6: ADVERSE DRUG REACTIONS (ADRS)

- Eight questions (2 marks each) which will be based on common adverse effects in order that you do not need to repeatedly refer to the BNF.
- There will be two questions from each subtype (A–D).
- You will have a list of five answer options to choose from.
- **You will be expected to identify:**
  - Likely adverse reactions and their causative agents
  - Potentially dangerous (black dot) interactions
- You will need to decide on the **best management approach** as a result of a given adverse reaction. This may include:
  - Administering a second agent to counteract the adverse effect (where appropriate to do so)
  - Discontinuing a given causative agent (drug or fluid)
  - Reducing a dose or rate (if infusion related) or frequency
  - Gradual withdrawal (e.g. benzodiazepines)
  - Avoiding a given interaction by choosing a more suitable drug

ADR QUESTION SUBTYPES AND SOME EXAMPLES

Type A	Type B	Type C	Type D
Identify the most likely effect of a specific drug	Identify the most likely medication to cause a given adverse reaction (or presentation)	Identify the drug most likely to be clinically important in a given presentation resulting from a potential interaction	Identify the most appropriate course of action for a given presentation or adverse reaction
Dry cough with ACEIs	Renal impairment (with nephrotoxic drugs)	Drug interactions such as:	Adverse events include:
Flushing and oedema with CCBs		Warfarin–statins	Acute anaphylactic reactions
Headache with nitro-vasodilators	Hepatic impairment (with hepatotoxic drugs)	NSAIDs–ACEIs	
Hypokalaemia with beta-2 agonists		Enzyme inducers and inhibitors (see below)	Excessive anti-coagulation
GI bleeding with NSAIDs	Hypokalaemia (with some diuretics, steroids and beta-2 agonists)		Drug-induced hypoglycaemia
Respiratory depression with opioids			Diuretic-induced dehydration
AKI with aminoglycosides	Urinary retention (with anti-muscarinic type agents)		

LIVER ENZYME INDUCERS AND INHIBITORS

- Enzyme inhibitors act quite quickly, usually within 24 hours.
- Enzyme inducers take longer to act, usually from 1 to 4 weeks.

Inhibitors	Inducers
Alcohol (acute)	Alcohol (chronic)
Amiodarone	Barbiturates
Cimetidine	Carbamazepine
Ciprofloxacin	Phenytoin
Erythromycin	Rifampicin
Isoniazid	Sulfonylureas
Ketoconazole	
Omeprazole	
Sodium valproate	
Sulfonamides	

As a general rule:

- Inhibitors will inhibit hepatic CYP450 iso-enzyme activity, thus leading to an increase in the amount of interacting drug (as it is not fully metabolized by a given CYP450 pathway).
- Inducers will induce hepatic CYP450 iso-enzyme activity, thus leading to a decrease in the amount of interacting drug (as it is metabolized more readily).

SECTION 7: DRUG MONITORING

- Eight questions (2 marks each).
- You will need to decide on how to monitor the effects of medicines in order to assess the effectiveness or lack thereof of a given medication.
- You will be given a scenario from which you will need to make judgements about assessing ongoing or soon-to-start treatment(s).
- You will be assessed on your ability to plan appropriate monitoring based on clinical parameters, examination findings and any investigations undertaken.
- Some example situations may include:
  - When to appropriately take blood levels for a narrow therapeutic index drug (e.g. gentamicin and vancomycin)
  - When to appropriately take blood levels for other relevant medication (e.g. certain anti-epileptics)
  - Timing of aspects of monitoring (e.g. peak vs trough level)
  - Monitoring while on amiodarone
  - Monitoring while on digoxin
  - Monitoring while on corticosteroids for asthma
  - Risk factors and monitoring with oral contraceptives
  - Use of drugs in hyperthyroidism (e.g. carbimazole)

SOME COMMON THERAPEUTIC DRUG MONITORING (TDM) LEVELS

Drug	Timing	Level
Carbamazepine	Trough (immediately pre-dose)	34–51 micromol/L
Digoxin	Trough (immediately pre-dose) **or** >6 hours post-dose	1–2 nanomol/L
Gentamicin	Peak (1 hour post-dose) **or** Trough (1 hour pre-dose)	**Peak:** 5–10 mg/L (or 3–5 mg/L in endocarditis) **Trough:** <2 mg/L (or <1 mg/L if endocarditis)
Lithium	Trough (12–18 hours after last dose)	0.5–1.2 mmol/L
Phenytoin	Anytime (if steady state reached)	**Total phenytoin:** 10–20 mg/L (40–80 micromol/L)
Sodium valproate	Trough (pre-dose)	50–100 mg/L (but poor evidence for taking a level as little correlation between dose and level)
Vancomycin	Trough (1 hour pre-dose)	10–15 mg/L
Theophylline	Trough (pre-dose)	55–110 micromol/L
Tobramycin	Peak (1 hour post-dose) **or** Trough (immediately pre-dose)	**Peak:** 5–10 mg/L (or 3–5 mg/L in endocarditis) **Trough:** <2 mg/L (or <1 mg/L if endocarditis)

SECTION 8: DATA INTERPRETATION

- Six questions (2 marks each).
- You will need to be able to interpret medical data and results of investigations based on ongoing drug therapy.
- You will be assessed on your ability to be able to make appropriate changes to a prescription based on your interpretation.
- **Courses of action available to you will include:**
  - Making no change
  - Changing a dose (either increasing or decreasing)
  - Discontinuing a medication
  - Initiating a new medication
- **Data that you may be asked to interpret include:**
  - Drug concentrations or levels
  - Blood gas readings
  - Blood count results (e.g. haemoglobin levels and white cell count)
  - Blood glucose readings
  - Urea and electrolyte values (U&Es)
  - Liver function tests (LFTs)
  - Kidney function values (e.g. glomerular filtration rate [GFR])
  - Lipid profile results (such as serum cholesterol)
  - Bone profile results (such as vitamin D levels)
  - Drug nomograms
  - Paracetamol poisoning treatment curve
  - Blood pressure readings

SOME COMMON DATA REFERENCE RANGES AND CAUSES OF DISTURBANCES

FBC	WCC	RBC	Hb	Plat	Neutrophils
Reference range	4–11	3.5–5.0 (F) 4.3–5.9 (M)	115–160 (F) 130–180 (M)	150–400	1.5–7
Units	x 10⁹/L	x 10¹²/L	g/L	x 10⁹/L	x 10⁹/L
Possible causes (↑)	Infection Leukaemia/lymphoma Drugs (e.g. immunosuppressants, steroids) Pregnancy	Polycythaemia rubra vera Renal disease Chronic lung disease Liver disease	Polycythaemia rubra vera COPD Renal disease High altitude	Malignancy Splenectomy Infection Inflammation Bleeding disorders	Infection Pregnancy
Possible causes (↓)	Drugs (e.g. chemotherapy drugs, carbamazepine, carbimazole) Immune disorders	Anaemia (microcytic, normocytic, macrocytic)	Anaemia (microcytic, normocytic, macrocytic) Bleeding Haemoglobinopathies	Autoimmune (e.g. ITP) Drugs (e.g. heparin) Bone marrow failure	Cancer Drugs (e.g. chemotherapy drugs, carbamazepine, carbimazole) Physiological make-up (African-Caribbean) Immune disorders

U&Es	Na	K	Urea	Cr	Mg
Reference range	137–144	3.5–4.9	2.5–7.0	60–110	0.75–1.05
Units	mmol/L	mmol/L	mmol/L	micromol/L	mmol/L
Possible causes (↑)	Burn states Dehydration states Diabetes insipidus Excess intake or excessive fluid replacement with sodium chloride 0.9%	Diabetic ketoacidosis Drugs (e.g. potassium-sparing diuretics, ACEIs, potassium supplements) Excess or inappropriate potassium replacement therapy Haemolysed blood sample Renal conditions (e.g. tubular nephropathy)	GI bleed Dehydration Hypertensive states Renal disease states	Kidney injury Dehydration Drugs (e.g. aminoglycosides)	Alcohol use Diarrhoea Drugs (e.g. diuretics) Malabsorption states Renal conditions (e.g. tubular necrosis)
Possible causes (↓)	Functional disorders (Addison's, cardiac, renal, hepatic, SIADH, hypothyroidism) Drugs (e.g. antidepressants, diuretics and carbamazepine) Diarrhoea/vomiting Fluid replacement therapy with a sodium deficit Hyperlipidaemia	Drugs (e.g. beta-agonists, diuretics, insulin) Lack of or insufficient replacement Diarrhoea/vomiting Renal acidosis	Pregnancy Muscle wasting states	Pregnancy	Drug misuse (e.g. antacids, laxatives) Renal failure

LFTs	ALT	ALP	Total Bilirubin	Total Protein	GGT	PT	INR
Reference range	5–35	45–105	<22	61–76	4–35 (F) <50 (M)	11.5–15.5	<1.4
Units	IU/L	IU/L	micromol/L	g/L	IU/L	seconds	(Ratio)
Possible causes (↑)	Liver damage (e.g. alcoholic liver disease, hepatitis, infections) Fatty liver (NAFLD) NASH Vitamin D deficiency Paget's disease Malignant liver lesions Drugs (e.g. NSAIDs, paracetamol overdose, antifungal agents)		Liver obstruction Jaundice Gilbert's syndrome	Malignancy states	Liver obstruction Alcohol abuse	Clotting factor deficiency states Vitamin K deficiency states Drugs (e.g. heparin, warfarin) Liver diseases (e.g. cholestasis, impairment)	–
Possible causes (↓)	–		–	Protein disorders malnutrition	–	–	–

Bone and lipid	Albumin	Corrected Calcium	Vitamin D	Phosphorus	Serum Cholesterol	Fasting Triglycerides
Reference range	37–49	2.20–2.60	>49.9	0.80–1.40	<5.2	0.45–1.69
Units	g/L	mmol/L	nanomol/L	mmol/L	mmol/L	mmol/L
Possible causes (↑)	–	Bone metastases Hyperparathyroidism Multiple myeloma Excess vitamin D	Excess vitamin D Hypoparathyroidism Renal disease		Hypothyroid states Fatty liver (NAFLD) Excessive dietary intake of fatty foods, red meat etc.	Alcohol misuse Diabetes Hereditary lipid disorders
Possible causes (↓)	Protein loss states (e.g. nephrotic syndrome) Malnutrition	Low levels of magnesium	Lack of exposure to direct sunlight Osteo-malacia Reduced dietary intake Rickets	Alcohol misuse Hyperpara-thyroidism Re-feeding syndrome	–	–

Haematinics	Serum Iron	Serum Ferritin	Serum Transferrin	Serum Vitamin B12	Serum Folate
Reference range	12–30	15–300	2.0–4.0	160–760	2.0–11.0
Units	micromol/L	microgram/L	g/L	nanogram/L	microgram/L
Possible causes (↑)	Sideroblastic anaemia Haemolysis	Acute illnesses	–	Leukaemia Liver disease Polycythaemia rubra vera Over-treated B12 deficiency	Excessive intake Pernicious anaemia Vegetarian diet
Possible causes (↓)	Iron deficiency anaemia GI blood loss Menorrhagia Malabsorption syndromes	Iron deficiency anaemia Haemolysis	Iron deficiency anaemia	Alcohol use Intrinsic factor deficiency (pernicious anaemia) Drugs (such as metformin) Low dietary intake Malabsorption syndromes Tuberculosis	Drugs (such as methotrexate, trimethoprim, co-trimoxazole) Low dietary intake Malabsorption syndromes Sickle cell disease Pregnancy states

Others	Fasting Glucose	HbA$_{1c}$	CRP	CK
Reference range	3.0–6.0	20–42 (4.0–6.0 %)	<5	24–170 (F) 24–195 (M)
Units	mmol/L	mmol/mol	mg/L	IU/L
Possible causes (↑)	Diabetes	Chronic diabetes	Infection Inflammation PMR GCA Malignancy states	Drugs (daptomycin, statins) Muscle disorders (e.g. dystrophy, rhabdomyolysis) Physiological (African-Caribbean) Diabetic finger pricking
Possible causes (↓)	Hypoglycaemic states Insulinoma	–	–	–

Acid-base	PO_2	PCO_2	pH	Lactate	Bicarbonate	Base Excess
Reference range	11.3–12.6	4.7–6.0	7.35–7.45	0.5–1.6	21–29	±2
Units	kPa	kPa		mmol/L	mmol/L	mmol/L
Possible causes (↑)	–	Hypo-ventilation Respiratory failure (T2)	Alkalosis	Anaerobic states Drugs (e.g. metformin)	Alkalosis	Alkalosis
Possible causes (↓)	Respiratory failure (T1)	Hyper-ventilation	Acidosis	–	Acidosis Diarrhoea states Renal impairment	Acidosis

INTERPRETING GLOMERULAR FILTRATION RATES

- GFR values are calculated using equations such as Cockcroft and Gault/ MDRD/CKD-EPI in adults, and the Schwartz equation in children. In general, the values are as tabulated below:

GFR range (mL/min/1.73 m²)	Comments
>90	Normal – Stage 1 if other evidence of kidney damage
60–89	Mild – Stage 2 if other evidence of kidney damage
30–59	Moderate – Stage 3; 3a if readings are chronically at 45–59, or 3b if readings are chronically at 30–44 (i.e. chronic kidney disease)
15–29	Severe – Stage 4
<15	End-stage renal failure (ESRF) – also called established renal failure

- Evidence of kidney damage may include among others proteinuria, haematuria, genetic renal disorders and radiologically confirmed abnormal kidney(s).

Cockcroft and Gault	Schwartz equation
eGFR in men (mL/min/1.73 m²) = {[140 – age (years) x mass (kg)] x 1.23/ [(serum Cr (micromol/L)]}[a]	GFR (mL/min/1.73 m²) = [36.2 × height (cm)/serum Cr (micromol/L)]

[a] In women, the result is multiplied by 0.85.

How to Use This Book

Students may find that they get the best use out of this book by two approaches; there will be those amongst you who prefer to start exam preparation well in advance, and this book will be suitable for you as it can be used as a learning tool for clinical pharmacology. You will find that the explanations provide you with a cue to read around the point being assessed, and will enable you to research the evidence base behind it. There will also be those amongst you who prefer to prepare in the last few weeks leading up the exam; this book can provide you with a format to test your knowledge and to accumulate key points in a rapid way.

One tip that most students find very useful in their final-year GP attachment is to sit with their GP tutor when they are signing off the repeat prescriptions, and being subjected to quick-fire viva-style questions pertaining to each prescription.

The authors have deliberately written the questions in the exam format with two sets of questions each of the same length as the exam itself, to allow you to have the option of completing each paper in exam conditions and then marking yourself at the end. Alternatively you may find it helpful to answer the question first and then check your answer by flicking to the back, then reading the explanation to reinforce your learning.

Students will also find that most of the questions are, in keeping with the PSA exam format, 'single best answer' with one option, usually out of five, being correct. There is occasionally more than one correct answer, and this will be specified in the question, as it is usually a particular question type. This has been shown to increase fairness of the exam compared to true/false exams by levelling the playing field with regard to a student's approach to risk. It has also been shown to be more helpful in discriminating between knowledgeable and unknowledgeable students in various medical examinations.

The authors have made every effort to cover the most commonly prescribed drugs in hospital and primary care settings, and have researched this by using literature that has facilitated this (2).

The authors have also targeted such resources as the SGUL 'Grey Book' and guidelines including NICE, BTS (British Hypertensive Society) and BHS (British Hypertension Society) to write questions that specifically address the curriculum that final-year students have to be familiar with. Students will also find that the explanations at the back of the book per question will act as a cue for them to read up on other relevant alerts and guidelines, such as the EMA (European Medicines Agency) or MHRA (Medicines and Healthcare Products Regulatory Agency) among other pharmacological texts.

The authors have also tried to ensure that the questions are of a similar standard to the PSA exam. We hope that this book will help you to calibrate yourself and have a better understanding of your current level of knowledge.

Although the authors have tried to minimize the degree of ambiguity in the answers, there may be occasions when more than one answer can be considered correct, in which case we do our best to address this in the explanation.

We hope that you enjoy using this book and find it to be a resource that is useful to you in your early careers as well as during further progression.

Abbreviations

A&E	Accident and Emergency department
ACEI	Angiotensin Converting Enzyme Inhibitor
AKI	Acute Kidney Injury
ALT	Alanine Aminotransferase
AMTS	Abbreviated Mental Test Score
ANC	Actual Neutrophil Count
AST	Aspartate Aminotransferase
AVF	Augmented Vector (lead)
AXR	Abdominal X-ray
Beta-HCG	Beta-Human Chorionic Gonadotrophin
BHIVA	British HIV Association
BHS	British Hypertension Society
BMI	Body Mass Index
BNF	British National Formulary
BNFC	British National Formulary for Children
BP	Blood Pressure
BTS	British Thoracic Society
CCB	Calcium Channel Blocker
CCF	Congestive Cardiac Failure
CCG	Clinical Commissioning Group
CHD	Chronic Heart Disease
CK	Creatine Kinase
CKD	Chronic Kidney Disease
CKD-EPI	Chronic Kidney Disease Epidemiology Collaboration
CMHT	Community Mental Health Team
CMV	Cytomegalovirus
COCP	Combined Oral Contraceptive Pill
COPD	Chronic Obstructive Pulmonary Disease
Cr	Creatinine
CRP	C-Reactive Protein
CT	Computed Tomography
CVA	Cerebrovascular Accident
CXR	Chest X-Ray
DCT	Distal Convoluted Tubule
DH	Drug History

DRESS	Drug Reaction with Eosinophilia and Systemic Symptoms
DVT	Deep Venous Thrombosis
eBNF	Electronic British National Formulary
EBV	Epstein–Barr Virus
ECG	Echocardiogram
ED	Emergency Department
eGFR	Estimated Glomerular Filtration Rate
EMA	European Medicines Agency
ENT	Ear, Nose and Throat
EPAU	Emergency Pregnancy Assessment Unit
EQUIP	Errors – Questioning Undergraduate Impact on Prescribing
FBC	Full Blood Count
FH	Family History
G#P#	Gravida #, Para # (i.e. number of pregnancies, number of live births)
GCA	Giant Cell Arteritis
GCS	Glasgow Coma Scale
GFR	Glomerular Filtration Rate
GGT	Gamma-Glutamyl Transpeptidase
GI	Gastro-Intestinal
GMC	General Medical Council
GORD	Gastro-Oesophageal Reflux Disease
GP	General Practitioner
GUM	Genito-Urinary Medical
Hb	Haemoglobin
HDU	High-Dependency Unit
HIV	Human Immunodeficiency Virus
HRT	Hormone Replacement Therapy
HS	Heart Sounds
IBS	Irritable Bowel Syndrome
INR	International Normalized Ratio
ITP	Idiopathic Thrombocytopenic Purpura
IV	Intravenous
JVP	Jugular Venous Pressure
LFTs	Liver Function Tests
LMP	Last Menstrual Period
MAOI	Monoamine Oxidase Inhibitor
MCMA	Monochorionic Monoamniotic Twins
MDRD	Modification of Diet in Renal Disease
MHRA	Medicines and Healthcare products Regulatory Agency
MI	Myocardial Infarction
mmHg	Millimetres of Mercury
MMR	Measles-Mumps-Rubella vaccine

MSU	Midstream Urine
NAFLD	Non-Alcoholic Fatty Liver Disease
NASH	Non-Alcoholic Steatohepatitis
NICE	National Institute of Health and Care Excellence
NICU	Neonatal Intensive Care Unit
NKDA	No Known Drug Allergies
NPIS	National Poisons Information Service
NPSA	National Patient Safety Agency
NPV	Negative Predictive Value
NSAID	Non-Steroidal Anti-Inflammatory Drug
OCP	Oral Contraceptive Pill
PCA	Patient Controlled Analgesia
PHQ-9	Patient Health Questionnaire
PID	Pelvic Inflammatory Disease
PMH	Past Medical History
PMR	Polymyalgia Rheumatica
PO	Per Oral
POP	Progestogen-Only Pill
PRN	*Pro Re Nata*, 'as the occasion arises'
PSA	Prescribing Safety Assessment
PT	Prothrombin Time
PTH	Parathyroid Hormone
PVD	Peripheral Vascular Disease
QOF	Quality Outcomes Framework
RR	Respiratory Rate
RTA	Road Traffic Accident
SCRIPT	Standard Computerised Revalidation Instrument for Prescribing and Therapeutics
SH	Social History
SIADH	Syndrome of Inappropriate Antidiuretic Hormone Secretion
SIGN	Scottish Intercollegiate Network
SNRI	Serotonin–Norepinephrine Reuptake Inhibitor
SSRI	Serotonin Selective Reuptake Inhibitor
STAT	Immediately
STI	Sexually Transmitted Infection
TA	Transabdominal
TB	Tuberculosis
TDM	Therapeutic Drug Monitoring
TENS	Transcutaneous Electrical Nerve Stimulation
THR	Total Hip Replacement
TOP	Termination of Pregnancy
TV	Transvaginal
U&Es	Urea and Electrolytes

UPSI	Unprotected Sexual Intercourse
URTI	Upper Respiratory Tract Infection
USS	Ultrasound Scan
UTI	Urinary Tract Infection
VITAL	Virtual Interactive Teaching and Learning
VTE	Venous Thromboembolism
WCC	White Cell Count
WHO	World Health Organization

PSA – Paper One

PRESCRIBING (8 QUESTIONS – 10 MARKS EACH)

Q1. A mother presents to her general practitioner (GP) surgery with her 8-week-old child who weighs 4.2 kg as she is concerned he is not gaining weight. The child has been bringing up feeds, is irritable and has not been sleeping well recently. PMH: Premature baby (32/40 weeks); the mother has previously had a breastfeeding assessment. DH: Nil. SH: Nil.

On examination

Unsettled child, no dysmorphia, normal fontanelle, no signs of dehydration, no epigastric mass.

Prescribing request

Use the GP form below to write a prescription for ONE drug that needs to be initiated to help treat this child's condition.

Pharmacy stamp	Age D.o.B.	Title, forename, surname and address
Number of days' treatment N.B.: Ensure dose is stated		
Endorsements		
Signature of prescriber		Date

Q2. A 26-year-old woman presents to hospital for normal delivery of a healthy baby boy. Following delivery her BP increases and is consistently around 155/104 mmHg. PMH: Nil. DH: Nil. SH: Lives with husband in family home, is a non-smoker and has not had alcohol for the past 9 months. She plans to breastfeed her child.

Investigations

Na^+ 140 mmol/L (137–144), K^+ 3.7 mmol/L (3.5–4.9), urea 3.1 mmol/L (2.5–7.0), ALT 20 U/L (5–35), AST 25 U/L (1–31), ALP 93 U/L (45–105), urine dipstick – protein +, Hb – 113 g/L (115–165), platelets – 200 × 10^9/L (150–400), plasma urate – 474 mmol/L (0.19–0.36)

Prescribing request

Use the hospital regular medicines prescription chart below to write a prescription for ONE drug that will help to control this woman's blood pressure.

		Date →					
		Time ↓					
Drug (approved name)		6					
Dose	Route	8					
Prescriber (sign + print)	Start date	12					
		14					
Notes	Pharmacy	18					
		22					

Q3. A 35-year-old man presents to medical assessment unit with a likely streptococcal pneumonia. This is his first medical admission and he has no known drug allergies. He is given empirical intravenous benzylpenicillin and immediately develops facial swelling, inspiratory stridor and a widespread urticarial rash. PMH: Nil. DH: Nil. SH: Nil.

On examination
Temperature 37.0°C, HR 130/min and regular, BP 95/64 mmHg, JVP not seen RR 40/min, O_2 sat 98% on air, HS normal, chest sounds – stridor.

Investigations
Na^+ 140 mmol/L (137–144), K^+ 3.7 mmol/L (3.5–4.9), urea 9 mmol/L (2.5–7.0), Cr 85 micromol/L (60–110), CRP 111 (<5)
Cardiac monitor shows a sinus tachycardia.
CXR shows a right lower lobar consolidation.

Prescribing request
Use the hospital 'once only' medicines prescription chart below to write a prescription for ONE drug to treat this patient.

		ONCE ONLY MEDICINES					
Date	Time	Medicine (approved name)	Dose	Route	Prescriber (sign + print)	Time given	Given by

Q4. A 30-year-old woman presents to her GP surgery for review of her asthma. PMH: Asthma. DH: She normally uses a beclomethasone 200 microgram inhaler at a dose of 1 puff BD and uses salbutamol as required. At the last consultation 6 weeks previously, regular salmeterol was added. This helped initially; however she is still experiencing symptoms and requires regular use of salbutamol to control her cough and wheeze. SH: Nil.

On examination
On auscultation there is mild wheeze bilaterally.

Prescribing request
Use the GP form below to write a prescription for ONE drug that is recommended as an increase in her asthma therapy.

Pharmacy stamp	Age	Title, forename, surname and address
	D.o.B.	
Number of days' treatment N.B.: Ensure dose is stated		
Endorsements		
Signature of prescriber		Date

Q5. An 85-year-old female is currently an in-patient on the geriatric ward and has developed diarrhoea. She is awaiting discharge, having been treated for a chest infection for which she was admitted 10 days previously. Prior to admission she had received multiple antibiotic courses, and more recently she has completed a course of co-amoxiclav. PMH: She has suffered from osteoporosis. DH: Alendronic acid and calcium/ergocalciferol tablets.

On examination

Temperature 37.5°C, HR 95/min and regular, BP 120/78 mmHg. On palpation of the abdomen she is diffusely tender with no evidence of peritonism.

Investigations

Urea 6.7 mmol/L (2.5–7.0), Cr 90 micromol/L (60–110), WCC 17×10^9/L (4–11), CRP 150 (<5)
Clostridium difficile toxin – positive.
AXR shows undistended bowel loops with no free gas under the diaphragm.

Prescribing request

Use the hospital regular medicines prescription chart below to write a prescription for ONE drug that will help to treat this woman's *C. difficile* infection.

		Date →					
		Time ↓					
Drug (approved name)		6					
Dose	Route	8					
Prescriber (sign + print)	Start date	12					
		14					
Notes	Pharmacy	18					
		22					

Q6. A 5-year-old child presents with his mum to the emergency department complaining of a 3 days history of ear-ache with accompanying fever. He has not vomited. His mum reports that his appetite is reduced and he is very irritable. PMH: He has atopic eczema. DH: He normally uses emollients and topical steroids as required. **Allergies:** Nut allergy only. SH: He lives with his parents and two siblings.

On examination

Temperature 38.5°C, HR 100/min, no rash or neck stiffness, negative Kernig's sign, normal chest and abdominal exam, negative urine dipstick.

Auroscope exam reveals a left red bulging tympanic membrane. Other important findings include a tender mastoid process.

Prescribing request

Use the hospital regular medicines prescription chart below to write a prescription for ONE drug that will help to treat his symptoms.

		Date →					
		Time ↓					
Drug (approved name)		6					
Dose	Route	8					
Prescriber (sign + print)	Start date	12					
		14					
Notes	Pharmacy	18					
		22					

Q7. A 33-year-old woman of 9 weeks' gestation presents to the emergency department complaining of severe nausea and vomiting with inability to tolerate oral fluids. She is G2 P1. She was given oral promethazine by her GP 24 hours ago. She had a 6-week scan due to excessive fatigue which revealed she had a twin pregnancy. PMH: Nil. DH: Folic acid. SH: She lives with her partner and 16-month-old son.

On examination
Temperature 36°C, HR 100/min and regular, BP 106/63 mmHg, O_2 sat 96% on air, abdominal examination normal, urine dipstick – ketones ++.

Investigations
Na^+ 137 mmol/L (137–144), K^+ 3.3 mmol/L (3.5–4.9), urea 3.2 mmol/L (2.5–7.0), Cr 60 micromol/L (60–110), eGFR 55 mL/min/1.73 m^2 (>60) ECG shows no effects of hypokalaemia.

Prescribing request
Use the hospital regular medicines prescription chart below to write a prescription for ONE drug that will help to treat her nausea.

		Date →						
		Time ↓						
Drug (approved name)		6						
Dose	Route	8						
Prescriber (sign + print)	Start date	12						
		14						
Notes	Pharmacy	18						
		22						

Q8. An 84-year-old woman presents to the emergency department complaining of unilateral headache and gripping pain in her shoulder and hips. PMH: Osteoarthritis. DH: She normally takes co-codamol, naproxen and omeprazole. SH: She lives alone.

On examination

Temperature 37°C, HR 82/min and regular, BP 138/85 mmHg, JVP unraised, RR 16/min, O$_2$ sat 96% on air, HS normal, chest sounds – bi-basal scattered crepitations, weight – 60 kg.

Other important observations are that she has tenderness over her left temporal artery, she cannot abduct her arms and she cannot stand from a chair.

Investigations

Na$^+$ 135 mmol/L (137–144), K$^+$ 3.5 mmol/L (3.5–4.9), urea 5.5 mmol/L (2.5–7.0), Cr 71 micromol/L (60–110), eGFR 68 (>60), ESR 105 mm/1st h (<20), CRP 97 (<5)

ECG normal.

CXR shows nothing of note.

Prescribing request

Use the hospital regular medicines prescription chart below to write a prescription for ONE drug that will help to treat her symptoms.

		Date →					
		Time ↓					
Drug (approved name)		6					
Dose	Route	8					
Prescriber (sign + print)	Start date	12					
		14					
Notes	Pharmacy	18					
		22					

PRESCRIPTION REVIEW (8 QUESTIONS – 4 MARKS EACH)

Q1. A 62-year-old woman presents to her GP for a medication review and is also complaining of a dry cough. PMH: She has suffered from angina, hypertension, CVA, psoriatic arthritis and diabetes. DH: She normally takes simvastatin, lisinopril, aspirin, carvedilol, verapamil, clopidogrel, folic acid, lansoprazole, metformin, methotrexate and gliclazide. SH: She lives alone.

Question A
Select the TWO prescriptions that have the potential to be a cause of her cough. Mark with a tick in column A.

Question B
Select the TWO prescriptions that are most likely to interact to cause her pre-syncope. Mark with a tick in column B.

CURRENT PRESCRIPTIONS					
Drug name	Dose	Route	Freq.	A	B
Aspirin	75 mg	Oral	Daily	☐	☐
Carvedilol	25 mg	Oral	Daily	☐	☐
Clopidogrel	75 mg	Oral	Daily	☐	☐
Folic acid	5 mg	Oral	Weekly	☐	☐
Gliclazide	80 mg	Oral	Twice daily	☐	☐
Lansoprazole	15 mg	Oral	Daily	☐	☐
Lisinopril	20 mg	Oral	Daily	☐	☐
Metformin	1 g	Oral	Twice daily	☐	☐
Methotrexate	10 mg	Oral	Weekly	☐	☐
Simvastatin	40 mg	Oral	Nightly	☐	☐
Verapamil	80 mg	Oral	Thrice daily	☐	☐

Q2. A 75-year-old woman presents to the medical assessment unit with melaena. PMH: Constipation, low mood, hypertension, type 2 diabetes, atrial fibrillation and stroke with residual epilepsy. She states that her atrial fibrillation is poorly controlled and, when her blood results return, they demonstrate an international normalized ratio (INR) of 9 (0.8–1.2) with haemoglobin of 80 g/L (115–165). DH: Her current regular medicines are listed below.

Question A
Select the ONE prescription that is most likely to interact with warfarin to raise the INR. Mark with a tick in column A.

Question B
Select the THREE prescriptions that are most likely to interact with digoxin. Mark with a tick in column B.

CURRENT PRESCRIPTIONS					
Drug name	Dose	Route	Freq.	A	B
Amlodipine	10 mg	Oral	Daily	☐	☐
Aspirin	75 mg	Oral	Daily	☐	☐
Bendroflumethiazide	2.5 mg	Oral	Daily	☐	☐
Digoxin	125 micrograms	Oral	Daily	☐	☐
Metformin	500 mg	Oral	12-hrly	☐	☐
Movicol®	1 sachet	Oral	12-hrly	☐	☐
Ramipril	5 mg	Oral	12-hrly	☐	☐
Sertraline	50 mg	Oral	12-hrly	☐	☐
Spironolactone	25 mg	Oral	Daily	☐	☐
Sodium valproate	1000 mg	Oral	12-hrly	☐	☐
Warfarin	2 mg	Oral	Daily	☐	☐

Q3. An 81-year-old man presents to the emergency department complaining of dizziness on standing. PMH: He has hypertension, chronic heart disease, hypothyroidism, iron deficiency anaemia and benign prostatic hypertrophy. DH: He normally takes amlodipine, ferrous fumarate, isosorbide mononitrate, levothyroxine, ramipril and tamsulosin.

On examination his blood pressure drops from 140/95 to 110/90 mmHg on standing. On review of his bloods, thyroid function tests continue to demonstrate hypothyroidism.

Question A
Select the THREE prescriptions that are most likely to be a cause of his postural hypotension. Mark with a tick in column A.

Question B
Select the ONE prescription that is most likely to be interacting with levothyroxine. Mark with a tick in column B.

CURRENT PRESCRIPTIONS					
Drug name	Dose	Route	Freq.	A	B
Amlodipine	10 mg	Oral	Daily	☐	☐
Ferrous fumarate	210 mg	Oral	Twice daily	☐	☐
Isosorbide mononitrate	25 mg	Oral	Twice daily	☐	☐
Levothyroxine	125 micrograms	Oral	Daily	☐	☐
Ramipril	10 mg	Oral	Daily	☐	☐
Tamsulosin	400 micrograms	Oral	Nightly	☐	☐

Q4. An 84-year-old woman is admitted to the acute medical unit with a sodium level of 157 mmol/L (137–144), having been transferred from the mental health unit where she was being treated for a manic episode. PMH: She has a history of bipolar disorder, COPD, ischaemic heart disease and congestive cardiac failure. DH: She normally takes the medications listed below.

On examination she is febrile at 38.1°C and is noted to have nystagmus and past-pointing.

Question A
Select the ONE prescription that is most likely to be contributing to the signs found on examination. Mark with a tick in column A.

Question B
Select the THREE prescriptions that are most likely to be contributing to the patient's hypernatraemia. Mark with a tick in column B.

CURRENT PRESCRIPTIONS					
Drug name	**Dose**	**Route**	**Freq.**	**A**	**B**
Aspirin	75 mg	Oral	Daily	☐	☐
Atorvastatin	40 mg	Oral	Daily	☐	☐
Bendroflumethiazide	2.5 mg	Oral	Daily	☐	☐
Bisoprolol	5 mg	Oral	Daily	☐	☐
Clopidogrel	75 mg	Oral	Daily	☐	☐
Furosemide	40 mg	Oral	Daily	☐	☐
Lithium	1.5 g	Oral	Daily	☐	☐
Ramipril	5 mg	Oral	Daily	☐	☐
Salbutamol 100 micrograms	2 puffs	INH	As required	☐	☐
Seretide® 250	2 puffs	Oral	Daily	☐	☐

Q5. A 53-year-old female presents to her GP surgery complaining of worsening symptoms of depression. PMH: Recurrent depression, paroxysmal atrial fibrillation, gastro-oesophageal reflux disease, hypothyroidism and chronic regional pain syndrome. DH: As listed below. SH: She lives with her husband who is an alcoholic and her son has recently been released from prison.

Question A
Select the ONE prescription that is most likely to contain a serious dosing error. Mark with a tick in column A.

Question B
Select the THREE prescriptions that are most likely to interact. Mark with a tick in column B.

CURRENT PRESCRIPTIONS					
Drug name	Dose	Route	Freq.	A	B
Amiodarone	200 mg	Oral	Twice daily	☐	☐
Amitriptyline	25 mg	Oral	Nightly	☐	☐
Citalopram	60 mg	Oral	Once daily	☐	☐
Levothyroxine	100 micrograms	Oral	Once daily	☐	☐
Omeprazole	10 mg	Oral	Once daily	☐	☐
Tramadol M/R	50 mg	Oral	Twice daily	☐	☐
Venlafaxine	150 mg	Oral	Once daily	☐	☐

Q6. A 28-year-old woman presents to your GP surgery requesting some advice on what medications she can use while breastfeeding. PMH: Hypertension and type 2 diabetes mellitus. DH: She normally takes medications as listed in the options below and has been recently started on an antibiotic for a urinary tract infection from hospital. SH: Nil.

Question A

Select the TWO prescriptions that are most likely to be safe to use while she is breastfeeding. Mark with a tick in column A.

Question B

Select the TWO prescriptions that should preferably be taken with food. Mark with a tick in column B.

CURRENT PRESCRIPTIONS					
Drug name	Dose	Route	Freq.	A	B
Aspirin (enteric coated)	75 mg	Oral	Daily	☐	☐
Ciprofloxacin	500 mg	Oral	12-hrly	☐	☐
Glibenclamide	5 mg	Oral	Daily	☐	☐
Lisinopril	10 mg	Oral	Daily	☐	☐
Metformin	1 g	Oral	8-hrly	☐	☐

Q7. A 45-year-old woman presents to the acute medical unit with complaining of polyuria, polydipsia and blurring of vision. PMH: She has a history of schizophrenia, recently diagnosed atrial fibrillation, hypertension, rotator cuff tear and multi-drug abuse and is currently being treated for a chest infection. DH: She normally takes the medications listed below. SH: She smokes 20 cigarettes a day and drinks one litre of whisky each evening.

The nurse measures her weight and height as 55 kg and 175 cm, respectively. Her blood glucose reading is 25 mmol/L.

Question A
Select the ONE prescription that is most likely to account for the presenting symptoms. Mark with a tick in column A.

Question B
Select the THREE prescriptions with an associated dosing error. Mark with a tick in column B.

CURRENT PRESCRIPTIONS					
Drug name	Dose	Route	Freq.	A	B
Clozapine	200 mg	Oral	Nightly	☐	☐
Codeine	30 mg	Oral	6-hrly	☐	☐
Digoxin	500 micrograms	Oral	Daily	☐	☐
Doxycycline	200 mg	Oral	Daily	☐	☐
Felodipine	10 mg	Oral	Daily	☐	☐
Ibuprofen	400 mg	Oral	8-hrly	☐	☐
Paracetamol	1 g	Oral	6-hrly	☐	☐
Vitamin B compound strong	1 tablet	Oral	Daily	☐	☐
Warfarin	2 mg	Oral	Daily	☐	☐

Q8. A 25-year-old Zimbabwean man presents to the genito-urinary clinic complaining of a rash and fever. His full blood count demonstrates an eosinophilia and his liver function tests are deranged. PMH: HIV, hypertension, gout and epilepsy. DH: His current regular medicines are listed below.

He is seen by a dermatologist who has diagnosed DRESS syndrome.

Question A
Select the ONE prescription that would be an inhibitor of cytochrome P450. Mark with a tick in column A.

Question B
Select the THREE prescriptions that are most likely to have caused the patient's rash, fever and eosinophilia. Mark with a tick in column B.

CURRENT PRESCRIPTIONS					
Drug name	**Dose**	**Route**	**Freq.**	**A**	**B**
Allopurinol	200 mg	Oral	Daily	☐	☐
Amlodipine	10 mg	Oral	12-hrly	☐	☐
Atazanavir/ritonavir	300 mg/100 mg	Oral	Daily	☐	☐
Carbamazepine	400 mg	Oral	12-hrly	☐	☐
Co-trimoxazole	480 mg	Oral	Daily	☐	☐
Emtricitabine	200 mg	Oral	Daily	☐	☐
Ramipril	5 mg	Oral	Daily	☐	☐
Tenofovir	245 mg	Oral	12-hrly	☐	☐

PLANNING MANAGEMENT (8 QUESTIONS, 2 MARKS EACH)

Q1. A 21-year-old man presents to the local walk-in centre complaining of a sore throat and a cough. PMH: He has suffered from recurrent tonsillitis. DH: Nil. **Allergies:** Penicillin. SH: Nil.

On examination

Temperature 38°C, tender cervical lymphadenopathy, enlarged tonsils with the right side larger than the left and whitish exudate on the tonsils noted.

Question

Select the most appropriate management option at this stage. Mark with a tick.

	MANAGEMENT OPTIONS	
A	Start the patient on a course of oral antibiotics for 7–10 days	☐
B	Advise the patient this is likely to be a self-limiting viral illness	☐
C	Refer the patient to the local emergency department to receive IV antibiotics from on-call ENT team	☐
D	Take a throat swab and ask for the GP to follow up the result in 3 days	☐
E	Arrange for a mono-spot blood test due to risk of Epstein–Barr virus	☐

Q2. A 60-year-old woman presents to the emergency department complaining of crushing central chest pain. PMH: Hypertension and type 2 diabetes mellitus. DH: She normally takes gliclazide, metformin and ramipril.

On examination

Temperature 36.6°C, HR 103/min and regular, BP 150/80 mmHg, JVP not raised, RR 20/min, O_2 sat 98% on air, HS pansystolic murmur, chest auscultation is unremarkable.

Investigations

Na^+ 141 mmol/L (137–144), K^+ 3.8 mmol/L (3.5–4.9), urea 6.9 mmol/L (2.5–7.0), Cr 100 micromol/L (60–110)
ECG shows ST segment elevation in leads II, III, aVF.
CXR normal.

Question

Select the most appropriate initial management option at this stage. Mark with a tick.

MANAGEMENT OPTIONS		
A	Aspirin	☐
B	Bisoprolol	☐
C	Clopidogrel	☐
D	Dalteparin	☐
E	Simvastatin	☐

Q3. A 35-year-old man presents to the endocrine clinic for follow-up of hypothyroidism complaining of polyuria, polydipsia and visual blurring. PMH: He suffers from hypothyroidism and his BMI is 33. DH: He normally takes levothyroxine.

Investigations

Thyroid function tests normal.
Fasting blood glucose 17 mmol/L (3–6).

Question

Select the most appropriate management option at this stage. Mark with a tick.

MANAGEMENT OPTIONS		
A	Repeat an oral glucose tolerance test for this patient	☐
B	Re-check the patient's fasting plasma glucose level in 4 weeks' time	☐
C	Commence an insulin regimen consisting of NovoMix® 30	☐
D	Take a blood sample to monitor urea and electrolyte levels	☐
E	Commence anti-diabetic medication in the form of metformin tablets	☐

Q4. A 90-year-old woman was admitted to the acute medical unit following a fall and has now developed a large haematoma on the flank on which she fell. PMH: She has a metallic aortic valve replacement. DH: She normally takes warfarin and her last INR was 2.1. SH: She lives alone and is independent.

On examination

HR 110/min and BP 88/54 mmHg. There is a large haematoma overlying her left buttock and thigh which appears to have expanded since admission.

Investigations

Haemoglobin 77 g/L (previously 110 g/L) (115–165), INR 6 (0.8–1.2), platelets 99×10^9/L (150–400)

Question

Select the most appropriate management option at this stage. Mark with a tick.

MANAGEMENT OPTIONS		
A	Continue warfarin (PO)	☐
B	Fresh frozen plasma (IV)	☐
C	Halt warfarin and commence VTE prophylaxis alone (SC)	☐
D	Pool of platelets (IV)	☐
E	Vitamin K (IV)	☐

Q5. A 19-year-old female presents to the emergency department complaining of acute severe pelvic pain, vomiting and mucopurulent discharge. Her last menstrual period was 8 days ago. PMH: She has no previous past obstetric or gynaecological history. DH: COCP (combined oral contraceptive pill). SH: She has had a recent change in sexual partner.

On examination
Temperature 38.5°C, HR 95/min and regular, BP 126/82 mmHg, suprapubic tenderness, no abdominal guarding or rebound tenderness. Pelvic exam reveals tenderness in both fornices and mild cervical excitation. Dipstick urine – negative.

Investigations
WCC 13.4×10^9/L (4.0–11.0), ESR 44 mm/1st h (<10), CRP 49 (<5)

Question
Select the most appropriate management option at this stage. Mark with a tick.

MANAGEMENT OPTIONS		
A	Send her home with a course of oral cefalexin	☐
B	Refer her for surgical assessment as query appendicitis	☐
C	Admit her for intravenous ceftriaxone, metronidazole and doxycycline	☐
D	Take swabs/urine samples and refer back to GP to chase the pathology report	☐
E	Refer her to the EPAU for a transvaginal US to exclude an ectopic pregnancy	☐

Q6. A 28-year-old woman presents to the local minor injuries unit complaining of a painful red, watery eye that feels as if there is something in it. She reports accidentally being poked in her eye with the branch of a tree while in the garden yesterday. She is able to look at lights and does not have any blurred vision. PMH: She normally wears contact lenses. DH: Nil. SH: None relevant.

On examination
The eye is diffusely red. There is no obvious foreign body in the eye.

Question
Select the most appropriate management option at this stage. Mark with a tick.

MANAGEMENT OPTIONS		
A	Apply an eye patch and review in one week	☐
B	Prescribe prophylactic broadspectrum topical antibiotics for 5 days	☐
C	Prescribe artificial tears due to the risk of a corneal scar	☐
D	Prescribe a one week course of local anaesthetic eye drops to take home	☐
E	Refer her to casualty to exclude a penetrating eye injury	☐

Q7. A 24-year-old man presents to the emergency department complaining of right upper quadrant pain. PMH: He has been feeling increasingly nauseous over the last 2 days and has been sick three times in the last 8 hours. DH: Nil regular but has been having co-codamol for last 24 hours. SH: Occasional smoker and drinker.

On examination

Temperature 37.5°C, HR 96/min and regular, BP 115/75 mmHg, O$_2$ sat 98% on air, abdomen is soft and tender.

Investigations

Na$^+$ 130 mmol/L (137–144), K$^+$ 3.2 mmol/L (3.5–4.9), urea 5.5 mmol/L (2.5–7.0), Cr 90 micromol/L (60–110), WCC 15.0 × 10^9/L (4.0–11.0), bilirubin 70 micromol/L (1–22), ALP 200 micromol/L (45–105), ALT 175 micromol/L (5–35)

Question

Select the most appropriate initial management option at this stage. Mark with a tick.

MANAGEMENT OPTIONS	
A	Initiate IV antibiotics to treat a possible infection	☐
B	Initiate IV cyclizine to alleviate emesis	☐
C	Initiate IV fluid management to rehydrate	☐
D	Initiate IV morphine for pain relief	☐
E	List the patient for a laparotomy	☐

Q8. A 45-year-old woman presents to the accident and emergency department with headache which was sudden in onset and severe. She describes it as being 'the worst headache I have ever had' and it is associated with marked photophobia. There is no history of a head injury. PMH: She has a history of depression for which she takes citalopram. FH: Her sister died from a subarachnoid haemorrhage.

On examination
Temperature 36.7°C, HR 85/min and regular, BP 120/78 mmHg, JVP not seen, RR 17/min, O_2 sat 100% in air. Remaining examination is unremarkable.

Investigations
Na^+ 137 mmol/L (137–144), K^+ 3.9 mmol/L (3.5–4.9), urea 5.5 mmol/L (2.5–7.0), Cr 62 micromol/L (60–110), CRP < 5
CT head (with contrast) – subarachnoid haemorrhage.

Question
Select the most appropriate initial management option. Mark with a tick.

	MANAGEMENT OPTIONS	
A	Dexamethasone	☐
B	Mannitol	☐
C	Metoprolol	☐
D	Nimodipine	☐
E	Tranexamic acid	☐

COMMUNICATING INFORMATION (6 QUESTIONS, 2 MARKS EACH)

Q1. A 28-year-old man presents with unresolving pain and erythema at a wound site following incision and drainage of a perianal abscess on the day surgery unit 2 days earlier. PMH: Chronic back pain and perianal abscess. DH: He is prescribed codeine, metronidazole and paracetamol.

Question

Select the most appropriate information option that should be communicated to the *patient* about the prescribed medication. Mark with a tick.

INFORMATION OPTIONS		
A	Codeine may cause diarrhoea	☐
B	Metronidazole is a painkiller	☐
C	Codeine can cause drowsiness	☐
D	Paracetamol should be taken only when needed	☐
E	It is safe to consume alcohol while on these drugs	☐

Q2. A 45-year-old woman who weighs 85 kg is seen in the gynaecology outpatient clinic with bouts of hot flushes, fatigue, urinary urgency and an irregular sleep pattern over the past 6 months. PMH: Nil. DH: Evening primrose oil. SH: Smokes 15 cigarettes per day; occasional social alcohol use.

Question

Select the most appropriate information option that should be communicated to this patient in order to help manage her condition. Mark with a tick.

INFORMATION OPTIONS		
A	Exercising late in the day will help to improve her sleep pattern	☐
B	Drinking more alcohol will help improve the hot flushes	☐
C	Taking regular exercise and losing weight may reduce the hot flushes	☐
D	Transdermal HRT will not be of use in helping control symptoms	☐
E	Having an irregular bedtime will help to improve her sleep pattern	☐

Q3. An 18-year-old woman presents to her local primary care walk-in-centre having consecutively missed two of her contraceptive pills. She is in the third week of her pack of pills. PMH: Nil. DH: Nil. SH: She smokes five cigarettes per day.

Question

Select the most appropriate information option that should be communicated to the patient. Mark with a tick.

	INFORMATION OPTIONS	
A	She should be advised to take emergency contraception now and adhere to extra precautions for 7 days	☐
B	She should be advised to follow the advice in her pill pack insert	☐
C	She should be advised to take 2 pills to cover her for the missed pills	☐
D	She should be advised to take 2 pills, to take extra precautions for next 7 days and to omit the next pill free week	☐
E	She should be advised to take 2 pills and advised to take extra precautions for 7 days	☐

Q4. A 1-year-old child is brought by her mother to her GP with an eczematous rash on her flexure surfaces and on her face, including around her eyes. PMH: She has suffered from eczema since 8 weeks of age. DH: Hydrocortisone 1% ointment, Diprobase® cream and Oilatum® bath additive. SH: Her mother bathes the child daily.

Question

Select the most appropriate information option that should be communicated to the mother. Mark with a tick.

	INFORMATION OPTIONS	
A	She should step up the steroid potency to a moderately potent product such as betamethasone 0.1% except for around the eyes	☐
B	The emollients should be applied frequently and in the same direction as hair growth	☐
C	She should bathe her child less frequently	☐
D	The area around the eyes can be treated with pimecrolimus	☐
E	The mother should be advised to step up the steroid potency to a moderate preparation such as betamethasone 0.1%	☐

Q5. A 15-year-old girl has been started on oral isotretinoin, having been referred to a dermatology clinic by her GP due to cystic-nodular acne. She has been asked to return to her GP surgery for monitoring and attends with her mother. She reports being sexually active. PMH: Nil. DH: COCP. SH: She lives with her parents.

Question
Select the most appropriate information option that should be communicated to the patient. Mark with a tick.

INFORMATION OPTIONS		
A	She must have a pregnancy test every month in the first 3 days of her cycle as part of a pregnancy prevention programme	☐
B	She needs to have regular blood tests for her lipids and LFTs	☐
C	She should alert the GP of onset of symptoms of depression	☐
D	She should be advised to stop it if her triglycerides increase	☐
E	Dry skin and dry mucus membranes are common side effects	☐

Q6. A 37-year-old woman presents to the ambulatory medical clinic complaining of tremor. On further questioning she reveals that this has commenced 8 weeks previously and has been associated with heat intolerance, sweating, insomnia and amenorrhoea. PMH: Nil. DH: Ferrous sulfate. SH: There is a family history of rheumatoid arthritis.

Investigations
Bloods are normal except for thyroid function tests which demonstrate TSH < 0.05 mU/L (0.5–5), and free T4 is 25 pmol/L (10–22).

She is diagnosed with hyperthyroidism and is commenced on carbimazole.

Question
Select the most appropriate information option that should be communicated to the patient. Mark with a tick.

INFORMATION OPTIONS		
A	Advise her to leave 4 hours between taking carbimazole and her ferrous sulfate	☐
B	Inform her that she should have repeat thyroid function testing in 1 week	☐
C	Counsel her that this medication commonly results in liver problems	☐
D	If she develops a sore throat then needs to seek medical attention	☐
E	She is also required to take regular folic acid supplementation	☐

CALCULATION SKILLS (8 QUESTIONS, 2 MARKS EACH)

Q1. An 85-year-old female is sent into the accident and emergency department by the staff at her nursing home, having developed confusion, vomiting, fever and rigors. A source of infection is not apparent and so the antibiotic protocol for 'sepsis of unknown source' is commenced. This suggests gentamicin.

You are required to prescribe a STAT dose of gentamicin. The hospital policy is for gentamicin to be given at 3 mg/kg provided that the creatinine clearance is greater than 20 mL/min/1.73 m².

The patient weighs 57 kg and her height is 160 cm.

Investigations
Urea – 11.5 mmol/L (2.5–7.0); Cr – 120 micromol/L (60–110)

Calculation
Using the equation below, what dose of gentamicin should be prescribed for this patient?

Estimated creatinine clearance (men) =
{[140 – age (years) × mass (kg)] × 1.23/[(serum Cr (micromol/L)]}
In women this result is multiplied by 0.85.
Write your answer in the box below.

Answer		Units:

Q2. A 33-year-old man requires adequate fluid replacement peri-operatively. You are instructed by your registrar to prescribe Hartmann's solution as fluid maintenance at a rate of 1.2 mL/kg/hr. The patient weighs 70 kg.

Calculation
What total volume, rounded to the nearest litre, over 24 hours should the patient be given?

Hartmann's solution comes in 500 mL or 1000 mL bags.
Write your answer in the box below.

Answer		Units:

Q3. A 12-year-old child is admitted to your paediatric ward with symptoms suggestive of eczema herpeticum. You are required to give a dose of intravenous aciclovir. The patient weighs 40 kg and is 150 cm tall.

Calculation
What dose should you prescribe?
Write your answer in the box below.

Answer		Units:

Q4. A 37-year-old man on an acute medical ward is due to be switched from his regular citalopram tablets which he has been taking at a dose of 20 mg daily to citalopram oral drops due to difficulty in swallowing.

Calculation

How many drops should you prescribe for the patient in order to get an equivalent dose to his tablets?

Write your answer in the box below.

Answer [   ] Units:

Q5. A 37-year-old homeless man weighing 55 kg with a PMH of acute alcohol withdrawal is to be discharged from the infectious diseases ward following admission for suspected tuberculosis. He has been lethargic for the past few months, with persistent cough, night sweats and apparent weight loss. Investigations confirm that he is culture positive and a QuantiFERON® -TB Gold test confirms the diagnosis. Due to compliance issues it is decided to start him on Voractiv® tablets.

Calculation

How many Voractiv tablets should be prescribed in total for the duration of the initial phase?

Write your answer in the box below.

Answer [   ] Units:

Q6. A 26-year-old woman is due for elective delivery and requires an infusion of zidovudine to prevent maternal–foetal transmission of HIV during delivery. Her booking weight is 78 kg and her current weight is 82 kg.

You are required to complete the infusion details in her care plan in readiness for the infusion. Your local guidelines suggest an intravenous loading dose of 2 mg/kg given over 1 hour, followed by a continuous intravenous infusion at 1 mg/kg until the umbilical cord is clamped. The patient's booking weight must be used for any calculations.

Calculation

What is the correct loading dose for this patient?

Write your answer in the box below.

Answer [   ] Units:

Q7. A 43-year-old female with bronchiectasis presents to your GP surgery after a recent hospital admission. She has been prescribed a reducing dose of prednisolone to help control her respiratory symptoms. Her hospital discharge letter states the following regime: 40 mg OM for 7/7, then 30 mg OM for 5/7, then 20 mg OM for 5/7, then 10 mg OM for 3/7, then 5 mg OM for 3/7, then stop. She has already been supplied 56 tablets from the hospital to help start her course.

Calculation

How many prednisolone 5 mg tablets should you prescribe in order for the patient to complete her course?

Write your answer in the box below.

Answer [ ]   Units: [ ]

Q8. An 84-year-old woman presents to the acute medical unit complaining of an erythematous rash overlying the posterior aspect of her neck and shoulders, and severe muscle pain. She is admitted and the results of investigations are consistent with dermatomyositis. She is commenced on 50 mg methylprednisolone intravenously due to nausea; however she is now feeling better and you are asked by your registrar to prescribe oral prednisolone instead.

You are given the following steroid, anti-inflammatory equivalences:

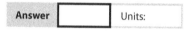

Prednisolone 5 mg ≡ Methylprednisolone 4 mg

Calculation

What total daily dose of oral prednisolone should be prescribed as an equivalent for the current dose of intravenous methylprednisolone?

Write your answer in the box below.

Answer [ ]   Units: [ ]

ADVERSE DRUG REACTIONS (8 QUESTIONS, 2 MARKS EACH)

Q1. A 54-year-old woman presents to her GP surgery complaining of urinary incontinence when she has an urge to pass urine. She has no symptoms of dysuria and she reports no leakage of urine when coughing, sneezing or standing up. PMH: She is G2P2 with two ventouse-assisted deliveries. DH: She normally takes levothyroxine 100 mg and omeprazole 10 mg. SH: She is a carer for her mother who has dementia.

On examination

She has no palpable bladder and no abnormal masses are elicited on abdominal examination. A urine dipstick is negative.

You decide to start her on tolterodine at a dose of 2 mg twice daily.

Question type A

Select the adverse effect that is most likely to be caused by this treatment. Mark with a tick.

ADVERSE EFFECT OPTIONS		
A	Agitation	☐
B	Dry mouth	☐
C	Nausea	☐
D	Sudden loss of vision	☐
E	Urinary retention	☐

Q2. A 42-year-old man presents to his GP surgery complaining of 12 kg weight gain in the past year. PMH: He has suffered from anxiety and depression for 1 year, atrial fibrillation, fatty liver and type 2 diabetes. DH: He normally takes digoxin, gliclazide, metformin, mirtazapine and temazepam. SH: He drinks 30 units weekly.

Question type B

Select the prescription that is most likely to be contributing to the weight gain. Mark with a tick.

PRESCRIPTION OPTIONS		
A	Digoxin	☐
B	Gliclazide	☐
C	Metformin	☐
D	Mirtazapine	☐
E	Temazepam	☐

Q3. A 15-year-old girl presents to hospital with a 3 month history of introverted behaviour, fatigue and abdominal pain. Upon investigation it is noted that she has severe anaemia and needs additional pain relief. She is reviewed by a psychiatrist and started on citalopram. PMH: Depression, hypo-parathyroidism and Ehlers–Danlos syndrome. DH: Adcal® D3 chewable tablets, alfacalcidol and paracetamol tablets.

Question type C

Select the prescription that is most likely to interact with citalopram and lead to an increased risk of bleeding. Mark with a tick.

PRESCRIPTION OPTIONS		
A	Alfacalcidol	☐
B	Adcal® D3	☐
C	Ferrous sulfate	☐
D	Ibuprofen	☐
E	Paracetamol	☐

Q4. A 26-year-old Asian man is transferred to the surgical assessment unit complaining of generalized abdominal pain which started from the right lower quadrant. He has been feeling sick since starting his new medication. PMH: Previous surgery for perforated ulcer 2 years ago. DH: He is on diclofenac 50 mg TDS and trimethoprim 200 mg BD for 3/7.

Question type D

Select the most appropriate option for the management of this adverse drug event. Mark with a tick.

MANAGEMENT OPTIONS		
A	Discontinue diclofenac	☐
B	Initiate lansoprazole	☐
C	Initiate ranitidine	☐
D	Discontinue trimethoprim	☐
E	Initiate Gaviscon® suspension	☐

Q5. A 55-year-old woman presents to a rheumatology outpatient clinic complaining of worsening joint pains. PMH: She has suffered from hypertension, gastro-oesophageal reflux disease and rheumatoid arthritis for 12 years. DH: She normally takes amlodipine, folic acid, ibuprofen (prn), methotrexate, paracetamol and ranitidine. SH: She lives alone, drinks less than 1 unit per week and has never smoked.

She is started on hydroxychloroquine by the rheumatologist.

Question type A
Select the adverse effect caused by this treatment that requires most monitoring in this patient. Mark with a tick.

PRESCRIPTION OPTIONS		
A	Arthropathy	☐
B	Keratopathy	☐
C	Neuromyopathy	☐
D	Photosensitivity	☐
E	Retinopathy	☐

Q6. A 43-year-old man presents to your surgery following a referral from his local pharmacist. He tells you he is getting regular headaches and flushing across his body which is causing him 'embarrassment'. PMH: Diabetes, hypertension, Raynaud's phenomenon and hypothyroidism. DH: Atenolol, levothyroxine, lisinopril, metformin and nifedipine.

Question type B
Select the prescription that is most likely to be contributing to the headaches and body flushing. Mark with a tick.

PRESCRIPTION OPTIONS		
A	Atenolol	☐
B	Levothyroxine	☐
C	Lisinopril	☐
D	Metformin	☐
E	Nifedipine	☐

Q7. A 63-year-old woman presents to her GP surgery complaining of muscle pain in her arms and legs. She has been recently discharged from hospital following type 2 respiratory failure and bilateral pneumonia. PMH: COPD, hypertension, type 2 diabetes and obesity. DH: Amlodipine 5 mg OM, clarithromycin 500 mg BD, gliclazide 80 mg BD, ramipril 5 mg OM, Seretide® '250' accuhaler, simvastatin 40 mg ON and tiotropium inhaler. SH: She lives alone as her husband passed away 2 years ago.

Question type C

Select the prescription that is most likely to interact with simvastatin and lead to an increased risk of rhabdomyolysis. Mark with a tick.

PRESCRIPTION OPTIONS		
A	Amlodipine	☐
B	Clarithromycin	☐
C	Gliclazide	☐
D	Ramipril	☐
E	Seretide	☐

Q8. An 18-year-old woman is referred to the medical assessment unit by her GP, following treatment for a urinary tract infection, with sudden-onset neutropenia, rash and liver dysfunction as confirmed by a blood test. A maculopapular eruption had developed into pustules over the preceding 3 days. PMH: Dysmenorrhoea. DH: Trimethoprim, paracetamol, ibuprofen and codeine. **Allergy:** Nil. SH: She works as a waitress.

Question type D

Select the most appropriate option for the management of this adverse drug reaction. Mark with a tick.

PRESCRIPTION OPTIONS		
A	Withhold all drugs until liver function returns to normal	☐
B	Stop ibuprofen as there is a risk of fluid retention	☐
C	Stop trimethoprim and manage the presenting symptoms	☐
D	Stop all drugs and allow the reaction to spontaneously resolve	☐
E	Prescribe intravenous fluconazole to treat neutropenic sepsis	☐

DRUG MONITORING (8 QUESTIONS, 2 MARKS EACH)

Q1. A 33/40-week-old neonate, one of monochorionic monoamniotic (MCMA) twins delivered by elective caesarean section 2 days ago and initially kept with the mother on the postnatal ward, is admitted on to the neonatal unit as she has over the last 24 hours become increasingly unsettled and steadily tachycardic, stopped passing stools and developed apnoeic episodes. She has been fed harvested colostrum, breast milk and formula since delivery. DH: She has been prescribed Abidec® 0.3 mL OD and caffeine citrate 20 mg OD. SH: Nil.

Question

Select the most appropriate monitoring option to assess the adverse effects of the caffeine treatment. Mark with a tick.

MONITORING OPTIONS		
A	Blood pressure	☐
B	Heart rate	☐
C	Therapeutic drug level	☐
D	Urinary output	☐
E	Weight gain/loss	☐

Q2. A 45-year-old man requires adequate fluid replacement following surgery. You prescribe Hartmann's solution as fluid maintenance.

Question

Select the most appropriate monitoring option to assess the beneficial effects of this treatment. Mark with a tick.

MONITORING OPTIONS		
A	Blood pressure	☐
B	Full blood count	☐
C	Oxygen saturations	☐
D	Respiratory rate	☐
E	Urea and electrolytes	☐

Q3. A 45-year-old woman presents to the accident and emergency department with confusion. She has not opened her bowels for a week. PMH: She has a history of alcoholic liver disease and a recent ultrasound demonstrated cirrhotic change. DH: She takes a regular vitamin B compound strong, thiamine and multivitamins. SH: She has not taken alcohol for 5 years.

On examination
Lying BP 132/73 mmHg, pulse 77/min; standing BP 130/75 mmHg, pulse 72/min.

Investigations
Hb stable, urea 6.0 mmol/L (2.5–7.0), Cr 71 micromol/L (60–110)

She is diagnosed with hepatic encephalopathy secondary to constipation and is commenced on regular lactulose, as well as thiamine replacement.

Question
Select the most appropriate monitoring option to assess the beneficial effects of this treatment. Mark with a tick.

MONITORING OPTIONS		
A	Blood pressure	☐
B	Oral intake	☐
C	Respiratory rate	☐
D	Stool chart	☐
E	Urine output	☐

Q4. A 55-year-old woman was admitted to the acute medical unit with neck stiffness, headache and fever. She is commenced on cefuroxime and a lumbar puncture is performed that demonstrates findings consistent with bacterial meningitis. She is commenced on ceftriaxone.

Question
Select the most appropriate monitoring option to assess the beneficial effects of this treatment. Mark with a tick.

MONITORING OPTIONS		
A	C-reactive protein	☐
B	White cell count	☐
C	Blood glucose	☐
D	Glasgow Coma Score	☐
E	Sensation to pin prick	☐

Q5. A 57-year-old man is newly initiated on digoxin at a dose of 125 micrograms once daily while in hospital for heart failure. He is discharged from hospital for routine primary care follow-up.

Question

Select the most appropriate monitoring option to assess the likely adverse effect of toxicity with this treatment. Mark with a tick.

MONITORING OPTIONS		
A	Blood pressure	☐
B	Potassium levels	☐
C	Pulse rate	☐
D	Respiratory rate	☐
E	Visual field tests	☐

Q6. A 39-year-old woman presents to her GP complaining of palpitations. PMH: She has suffered from depression for 4 years. DH: She normally takes venlafaxine. SH: She is a single parent who lives in social housing with her five children.

On examination

Pulse 80/min, regular; BP 139/85 mmHg.

Question

Select the most appropriate monitoring option to assess the effects of this treatment. Mark with a tick.

MONITORING OPTIONS		
A	Regular BP monitoring	☐
B	Ambulatory BP monitoring	☐
C	Regular FBC and U&Es	☐
D	Regular BP and ECG monitoring	☐
E	Regular blood and ECG monitoring	☐

Q7. An 18-year-old woman presents to the dermatology clinic with severe eczema which has required several courses of oral corticosteroids to control. She is commenced on azathioprine orally.

Question

Select the most appropriate monitoring option to assess the adverse effects of this treatment. Mark with a tick.

MONITORING OPTIONS		
A	Peak expiratory flow rate	☐
B	Full blood count monitoring	☐
C	Serum azathioprine concentration	☐
D	Urea and electrolytes	☐
E	Chest radiograph	☐

Q8. A 34-year-old woman diagnosed with bipolar disorder was started by the CMHT on Priadel® (lithium carbonate) tablets 6 months ago and was stabilized on a regular dose. She has been advised to see her GP for some blood tests to monitor this from now on.

Question

Select the most appropriate monitoring option to assess the adverse effects of this treatment. Mark with a tick.

MONITORING OPTIONS		
A	Lithium levels within 2 hours of a dose, every 6 months	☐
B	Renal function every 3 months, after initiation	☐
C	Thyroid function test annually	☐
D	Thyroid, renal and lithium levels every 6 months	☐
E	Lithium levels 12 hours after taking a dose, every 3 months	☐

DATA INTERPRETATION (6 QUESTIONS, 2 MARKS EACH)

Q1. A 67-year-old Pakistani man is advised to see his GP, having had an NHS Health check with the nurse. PMH: Hypertension. DH: He normally takes felodipine. FH: Unknown. SH: Smokes 15 cigarettes per day.

On examination
Height 173 cm, weight 90 kg, BP 158/96 mmHg.

Investigations
Serum cholesterol 6.3 mmol/L (<5.2), LDL 4.1 mmol/L (<3.36), HDL 0.9 mmol/L (>1.55), triglycerides 1.1 mmol/L (0.45–1.69) and HbA_{1C} 41 (>43)

Question
Select the most appropriate decision option with regard to the treatment of his cardiovascular disease based on these data. Mark with a tick.

DECISION OPTIONS		
A	Smoking cessation advice is the best advice for this man	☐
B	Advise diet and exercise and repeat check in 3/12 months	☐
C	Optimize the control of this gentleman's BP with anti-hypertensive therapy	☐
D	Commence this patient on anti-platelet therapy (i.e. aspirin)	☐
E	Commence this patient on anti-lipid therapy (i.e. a statin)	☐

Q2. A 33-year-old woman presents with right flank pain suggestive of acute pyelonephritis. On examination she has a temperature of 39.4°C, rigors, HR 160/min and regular, BP 105/70 mmHg. She is admitted to ward. PMH: She has been sick for the last few days since her last discharge for a urinary tract infection and has passed blood in her urine this morning.

Question
Select the most appropriate decision option with regard to the initial treatment of this woman based on the above data. Mark with a tick.

DECISION OPTIONS		
A	Arrange for a midstream urine test	☐
B	Prescribe an oral antibiotic	☐
C	Prescribe an intravenous antibiotic	☐
D	Referral to investigate any renal abnormality	☐
E	Referral back to primary care for management	☐

Q3. A 52-year-old woman presents to her GP surgery following a blood test due to symptoms of new-onset nausea and swelling of ankles. She has recently been started on ramipril. PMH: She has suffered from hypertension for 5 years and PVD. DH: She normally takes indapamide and amlodipine. SH: She is a widow of 3 years.

Investigations
K+ 4.2 mmol/L (3.5–4.9), Na+ 138 mmol/L (137–144), urea 9.4 mmol/L (2.5–7.0), Cr 110 micromol/L (60–90), eGFR 36 mL/min/1.73 m^2 (>60)
BP is 162/92.
Baseline eGFR was 58 mL/min/1.73 m^2.

Question
Select the most appropriate decision option with regard to the nausea and swelling of ankles based on the above data. Mark with a tick.

DECISION OPTIONS		
A	Stop the amlodipine	☐
B	Refer acutely to the local ED	☐
C	Stop the indapamide	☐
D	Treat with prochlorperazine	☐
E	Stop the ramipril	☐

Q4. A 33-year-old woman presents to hospital complaining of episodes of high blood pressure. Her last three readings over the past few days have been 160/110, 158/112 and 158/108 mmHg. PMH: She is of 33/40 weeks gestation and has no other history of note. DH: Nil. SH: Non-smoker and does not drink alcohol.

Question
Select the most appropriate treatment option with regard to the management of this woman's condition based on the above information. Mark with a tick.

DECISION OPTIONS		
A	Atenolol	☐
B	Enalapril	☐
C	Labetalol	☐
D	Methyldopa	☐
E	Nifedipine	☐

Q5. A 75-year-old man is referred to the acute medical clinic by his GP complaining of new-onset constipation and abdominal pain, and was found to have hypercalcaemia when the GP arranged blood tests. PMH: He has a history of osteoarthritis and vitamin D deficiency. DH: He normally takes Fultium® D3 (colecalciferol). SH: Current smoker of 10 cigarettes per day.

Investigations
Urea 6.7 mmol/L (2.5–7.0), Cr 101 micromol/L (60–110), corrected calcium 2.65 mmol/L (2.20–2.60), phosphate 1.6 mmol/L (0.8–1.4), PTH 0.7 pmol/L (0.9–5.4), ESR 3 mm/1st h (<10), Bence–Jones protein negative

Question
Select the most appropriate decision option with regard to management based on these data. Mark with a tick.

DECISION OPTIONS		
A	Initiate intravenous pamidronate	☐
B	Initiate magnesium glycerophosphate	☐
C	Withold Fultium D3	☐
D	Initiate Sandoz® Phosphate	☐
E	Initiate furosemide	☐

Q6. A 27-year-old primigravid African-Caribbean woman, of 28/40 gestation, presents to the antenatal clinic for gestational diabetes screening. On questioning she has had some symptoms of polyuria which she considers normal for pregnancy. PMH: Nil. DH: Nil. FH: NIDDM. SH: Nil.

Investigations
Fasting blood glucose 7.3 mmol/L (4.0–6.0), 2 hours post-glucose load 11.6 mmol/L (<11.0)

Question
Select the most appropriate decision option with regard to her blood glucose based on these data. Mark with a tick.

DECISION OPTIONS		
A	Advise she is pre-diabetic and needs blood glucose monitoring	☐
B	Advise she is diabetic and recommend dietary changes and exercise only	☐
C	Advise she is diabetic and start metformin	☐
D	Advise all of the above (points A–C)	☐
E	Advise she has gestational diabetes, start monitoring and consider treatment	☐

PSA – Paper Two

PRESCRIBING (8 QUESTIONS – 10 MARKS EACH)

Q1. An 80-year-old man presents to the accident and emergency department (A&E) with right lower leg cellulitis. PMH: He has a history of type 2 diabetes, ischaemic heart disease, chronic kidney disease and recurrent cellulitis. DH: His regular medications include gliclazide, metformin, aspirin and ramipril.

On examination
Temperature 36.7°C, HR 95/min and regular, BP 120/78 mmHg, JVP not seen, RR 17/min, O_2 sat 100% on air. The right lower leg is erythematous, warm, swollen and tender.

Investigations
Na^+ 141 mmol/L (137–144), K^+ 7.0 mmol/L (3.5–4.9), urea 5.0 mmol/L (2.5–7.0), Cr 65 micromol/L (60–110), CRP 111

Prescribing request
He has been given intravenous calcium gluconate by the registrar in A&E. Write a prescription for ONE further intravenous drug to treat this patient.

		INFUSION THERAPY							
Date	Start time	Infusion solution					Medicine added		Prescriber's signature	Given by
		Type/ strength	Volume	Route	Rate	Duration	Approved name	Dose		

Q2. An 85-year-old woman is brought into A&E by ambulance from her nursing home. The staff at the home have noticed that she has become increasingly confused over the past week and is now having fevers and foul-smelling urine. PMH: She has type 2 diabetes and osteopoenia. DH: She normally takes metformin, colecalciferol and alendronic acid.

On examination
Temperature 39°C, HR 92/min and regular, BP 120/93 mmHg, JVP not visible, RR 18/min, O_2 sat 99% on air, HS normal, chest sounds clear, weight 65.3 kg.

Investigations
Na^+ 145 mmol/L (137–144), K^+ 4.5 mmol/L (3.5–4.9), urea 19 mmol/L (2.5–7.0), Cr 170 micromol/L (60–110), eGFR 26 mL/min/1.73 m^2 (>60)
Urine dipstick: leucocytes and nitrites positive, sent for microscopy, culture and sensitivities.
CXR: No evidence of consolidation.

She is commenced on antibiotics for a urinary tract infection.

Prescribing request
Use the hospital regular medicines prescription chart below to write a prescription for ONE drug that will help to prevent venous thromboembolism in this woman.

		Date →					
		Time ↓					
Drug (approved name)		6					
Dose	Route	8					
Prescriber (sign + print)	Start date	12					
		14					
Notes	Pharmacy	18					
		22					

Q3. A 23-year-old man presents to the emergency department having been found collapsed at home by a friend. **PMH:** He has suffered from depression and substance misuse in the past. **DH:** He takes methadone and amitriptyline. **SH:** He drinks 35 units of alcohol a week and has a history of multiple substance misuse.

On examination

Temperature 36.1°C, HR 65/min and regular, BP 100/63 mmHg, RR 8/min, O_2 sat 92% on air, chest sounds clear. GCS (E1 V2 M4). Pupils are equal and 1 mm bilaterally.

Investigations

ECG shows sinus rhythm with narrow QRS.

Prescribing request

Use the hospital 'once only' medicines prescription chart below to write a prescription for ONE drug that will help to treat the patient's current condition.

ONCE ONLY MEDICINES							
Date	Time	Medicine (approved name)	Dose	Route	Prescriber (sign + print)	Time given	Given by

Q4. A 21-year-old woman presents to a family planning clinic requesting emergency contraception. She has not been using any form of hormonal contraception and she reports that the condom split on this occasion. Her LMP was 2 weeks ago. The unprotected sexual intercourse (UPSI) was the night before. PMH: Nil. DH: Nil. SH: She had a termination of pregnancy (TOP) 2 years ago.

On examination
BP 122/72 mmHg.

Prescribing request
Use the general practitioner (GP) form below to write a prescription for ONE drug that will help to prevent a pregnancy.

Pharmacy stamp	Age	Title, forename, surname and address
	D.o.B.	
Number of days' treatment N.B.: Ensure dose is stated		
Endorsements		
Signature of prescriber		Date

Q5. A 44-year-old woman presents to her GP complaining of mucopurulent nasal discharge and facial pain. The symptoms developed 3 days ago following an URTI that started 10 days previously. **PMH:** Nil. **DH:** Nil. **Allergies:** Nil. **SH:** Nil.

On examination
Temperature 38.2°C. Patient has facial tenderness on palpation over the frontal and maxillary sinuses.

Prescribing request
Use the GP form below to write a prescription for ONE drug that will help to treat the woman's acute sinusitis.

Pharmacy stamp	Age	Title, forename, surname and address
	D.o.B.	
Number of days' treatment N.B.: Ensure dose is stated		
Endorsements		
Signature of prescriber		Date

Q6. A mother presents with her 3-year-old son weighing 15 kg to her GP surgery following a visit to the paediatric emergency department a few days earlier. Her son has a skin rash to the face and upper torso which has a characteristic yellow crusty edge. PMH: The child has suffered from eczema for the last year and is allergic to penicillin. The emergency department has undertaken a skin swab and advised the GP to review. DH: Emollient and steroid creams. SH: Lives with parents; father suffers from eczema.

On examination
Temperature 37.4°C, HR 90/min and regular, BP 110/70 mmHg, RR 20/min, O$_2$ sat 99% in air.

Investigations
The GP views the child's skin swab results which show moderate growth of *Staphylococcus aureus*.

Prescribing request
Use the GP form below to write a prescription for ONE drug that needs to be initiated to help treat this skin condition.

Pharmacy stamp	Age	Title, forename, surname and address
	D.o.B.	
Number of days' treatment N.B.: Ensure dose is stated		
Endorsements		
Signature of prescriber		Date

Q7. A 27-year-old woman presents to her GP practice complaining of severe constipation. She is 33 weeks pregnant and tells you she has had difficulty with her bowel movements virtually every day of the week for the past few weeks. She has previously received dietetic referral and has increased her fluid intake as well as consumption of food and fruit rich in fibre. PMH: Nil. DH: Nil. SH: Non-smoker and non-alcoholic.

On examination
Temperature 37.4°C, HR 80 bpm, regular BP 120/82 mmHg. She has no 'red flag' signs.

Prescribing request
Use the GP prescription form below to write a prescription for ONE drug that will help to relieve this woman's constipation.

Pharmacy stamp	Age	Title, forename, surname and address
	D.o.B.	
Number of days' treatment N.B.: Ensure dose is stated		
Endorsements		
Signature of prescriber		Date

Q8. A 53-year-old man presents to the emergency department with central chest pain radiating to his jaw. He describes the pain as being tightness in his chest which was brought on by exertion. He is visibly sweating from his forehead. He tells you he has chewed an aspirin tablet while on his way to the hospital. PMH: Suspected acute coronary syndrome which is still under investigation. DH: Nil. SH: Ex-smoker, drinks approximately 10 units of alcohol per week.

Prescribing request

Use the hospital 'once only' medicines prescription chart below to prescribe ONE drug that needs to be given immediately to help with his chest complaint.

ONCE ONLY MEDICINES

Date	Time	Medicine (approved name)	Dose	Route	Prescriber (sign + print)	Time given	Given by

PRESCRIPTION REVIEW (8 QUESTIONS – 4 MARKS EACH)

Q1. A 55-year-old man was admitted to the coronary care unit with chest pain and shortness of breath. He underwent primary coronary intervention in the form of angioplasty and stent insertion to the left anterior descending artery. The following day his bloods demonstrate acute kidney injury [Cr 200 micromol/L (90 on admission), urea 19 mmol/L (6 on admission), eGFR 35 mL/min/1.73m^2]. **PMH:** He has suffered from obesity, type 2 diabetes mellitus, hypertension and hypercholesterolaemia. Prior to admission he was smoking 30 cigarettes per day. His current regular medicines are listed below.

Question A
Select the ONE prescription that is most likely to interact with clopidogrel to give an adverse effect. Mark with a tick in column A.

Question B
Select the THREE prescriptions that would be best to withhold in the context of acute kidney injury. Mark with a tick in column B.

CURRENT PRESCRIPTIONS					
Drug name	**Dose**	**Route**	**Freq.**	**A**	**B**
Aspirin	75 mg	Oral	Daily	☐	☐
Atorvastatin	40 mg	Oral	Daily	☐	☐
Bisoprolol	2.5 mg	Oral	Daily	☐	☐
Clopidogrel	75 mg	Oral	Daily	☐	☐
Fondaparinux	2.5 mg	SC	Daily	☐	☐
Furosemide	40 mg	Oral	Daily	☐	☐
Metformin	1 g	Oral	12-hrly	☐	☐
Omeprazole	40 mg	Oral	Daily	☐	☐
Ramipril	2.5 mg	Oral	Daily	☐	☐

Q2. A 77-year-old man presents to the ambulatory medical clinic complaining of a blistering erythematous rash. He has been treated over the past 3 days with amoxicillin for a chest infection by his GP. PMH: He has a history of ischaemic heart disease, congestive cardiac failure, hypothyroidism and resistant generalized epilepsy, for which his treatment has recently been escalated. DH: NKDA; his current regular medicines are listed below.

Investigation
INR 8.2 (0.8–1.2)

Question A
Select the THREE prescriptions that are most likely to interact with warfarin. Mark with a tick in column A.

Question B
Select the ONE drug that is most likely to have caused the rash. Mark with a tick in column B.

CURRENT PRESCRIPTIONS					
Drug name	Dose	Route	Freq.	A	B
Amoxicillin	250 mg	Oral	8-hrly	☐	☐
Aspirin	75 mg	Oral	Daily	☐	☐
Atorvastatin	40 mg	Oral	Daily	☐	☐
Bisoprolol	5 mg	Oral	Daily	☐	☐
Furosemide	40 mg	Oral	Twice daily	☐	☐
Lamotrigine	50 mg	Oral	12-hrly	☐	☐
Levothyroxine	125 micrograms	Oral	Daily	☐	☐
Omeprazole	40 mg	Oral	Daily	☐	☐
Ramipril	2.5 mg	Oral	Daily	☐	☐
Sodium valproate	1 g	Oral	12-hrly	☐	☐
Warfarin	6 mg	Oral	Daily	☐	☐

Q3. A 21-year-old Asian woman presents to her GP surgery for a routine pill check. She has been on the COCP for 2 years. PMH: She suffers from epilepsy, acne vulgaris, onychomycosis, hypothyroidism and GORD. DH: She takes carbamazepine, rifabutin, lymecycline, griseofulvin, levo-thyroxine and omeprazole. SH: Her mother was recently diagnosed with reactivated old TB. She lives with her husband.

Her current regular medicines are listed.

Question A
Select the THREE prescriptions that are most likely to interact. Mark with a tick in column A.

Question B
Select the TWO to THREE prescriptions that contains a serious dosing error. Mark with a tick in column B.

CURRENT PRESCRIPTIONS					
Drug name	Dose	Route	Freq.	A	B
Carbamazepine	200 mg	Oral	Twice daily	☐	☐
Griseofulvin	500 mg	Oral	Once daily	☐	☐
Levothyroxine	100 micrograms	Oral	Once daily	☐	☐
Lymecycline	408 mg	Oral	Twice daily	☐	☐
Omeprazole	10 mg	Oral	Once daily	☐	☐
Rifabutin	300 mg	Oral	Once daily	☐	☐
Bendroflumethiazide	2.5 mg	Oral	Once daily	☐	☐

Q4. An 84-year-old man is referred to the on-call 'care of older people team' with symptoms of dizziness. He has had a recent set of blood tests from his GP surgery that are available for you to review. PMH: Diabetes type 2, epilepsy, depression and hypertension. SH: Non-smoker, alcohol 20 units per week.

Question A
Select ONE prescription that is most likely to be the cause of his dizziness. Mark with a tick in column A.

Question B
Select THREE prescriptions that are most likely to be contributing to his low sodium. Mark with a tick in column B.

CURRENT PRESCRIPTIONS					
Drug name	Dose	Route	Freq.	A	B
Bendroflumethiazide	2.5 mg	Oral	Daily	☐	☐
Carbamazepine	400 mg	Oral	12-hrly	☐	☐
Fluoxetine	20 mg	Oral	Daily	☐	☐
Gliclazide	80 mg	Oral	Daily	☐	☐
Metformin	1 g	Oral	Twice daily	☐	☐
Ramipril	5 mg	Oral	Daily	☐	☐
Simvastatin	40 mg	Oral	Daily	☐	☐

Q5. A 52-year-old man presents to his GP for his medication review and is also complaining of an exquisitely painful and tender big toe. He has not had any trauma to his toe. PMH: Asthma, hypothyroidism, GORD, hypertension and CHD. DH: He normally takes amlodipine, aspirin, beclomethasone inhaler, bisoprolol, levothyroxine, omeprazole, ramipril and salbutamol inhaler. SH: None.

Question A
Select ONE prescription that is contraindicated. Mark with a tick in column A.

Question B
Select the TWO prescriptions that are most likely to be a cause of his symptoms of a painful big toe. Mark with a tick in column B.

CURRENT PRESCRIPTIONS					
Drug name	**Dose**	**Route**	**Freq.**	**A**	**B**
Amlodipine	10 mg	Oral	Daily	☐	☐
Aspirin	75 mg	Oral	Daily	☐	☐
Beclomethasone 50 microgram inhaler	2 puffs	INH	Twice daily	☐	☐
Bisoprolol	5 mg	Oral	Daily	☐	☐
Levothyroxine	100 mg	Oral	Daily	☐	☐
Omeprazole	10 mg	Oral	Daily	☐	☐
Ramipril	10 mg	Oral	Daily	☐	☐
Salbutamol 100 microgram inhaler	2 puffs	Oral	As required	☐	☐

Q6. A 62-year-old woman presents to her GP for her medication review and is also complaining of a dry tickly cough. PMH: She has suffered from angina, hypertension, CVA and diabetes. DH: She normally takes lisinopril, aspirin, carvedilol, verapamil, clopidogrel, lansoprazole, metformin and gliclazide.

Question A
Select the ONE prescription that is most likely to be a cause of her dry cough. Mark with a tick in column A.

Question B
Select the THREE prescriptions that are most likely to interact to cause her pre-syncope. Mark with a tick in column B.

CURRENT PRESCRIPTIONS					
Drug name	**Dose**	**Route**	**Freq.**	**A**	**B**
Aspirin	75 mg	Oral	Daily	☐	☐
Carvedilol	25 mg	Oral	Daily	☐	☐
Clopidogrel	75 mg	Oral	Daily	☐	☐
Gliclazide	80 mg	Oral	Twice daily	☐	☐
Lansoprazole	15 mg	Oral	Daily	☐	☐
Lisinopril	20 mg	Oral	Daily	☐	☐
Metformin	1 g	Oral	Twice daily	☐	☐
Simvastatin	40 mg	Oral	Nocte	☐	☐
Verapamil	80 mg	Oral	8-hrly	☐	☐

Q7. A 63-year-old man is due for a right THR. He presents to a pre-operative assessment clinic for review a week before the procedure. PMH: Type 2 diabetes mellitus, gastro-oesophageal reflux disease, heart failure and hypercholesterolaemia. DH: He normally takes medications as listed in the options below. SH: He lives alone and is an ex-smoker (quit 10 years ago).

Question A
Select the TWO prescriptions that are most likely to be stopped around a week prior to surgery. Mark with a tick in column A.

Question B
Select the TWO prescriptions that are to be omitted in this patient on the day of surgery. Mark with a tick in column B.

CURRENT PRESCRIPTIONS					
Drug name	Dose	Route	Freq.	A	B
Aspirin	75 mg	PO	Daily	☐	☐
Bisoprolol	5 mg	Oral	Daily	☐	☐
Bendroflumethiazide	2.5 mg	Oral	Daily	☐	☐
Gliclazide MR	30 mg	Oral	Daily	☐	☐
Lansoprazole	15 mg	Oral	Nightly	☐	☐
Metformin	850 mg	Oral	8-hrly	☐	☐
Ramipril	2.5 mg	Oral	Daily	☐	☐
Simvastatin	20 mg	Oral	Nightly	☐	☐
Spironolactone	25 mg	Oral	Daily	☐	☐

Q8. A 42-year-old woman presents to the psychiatric clinic for review of her depression. She has a history of dry eyes. On systems review she reports having black stools. PMH: She has suffered from ischaemic heart disease, osteoarthritis of the knees, depression, allergic rhinitis and vitamin D deficiency. DH: Her usual medications are listed below. SH: She lives alone.

Though haemodynamically stable she is found to have a microcytic anaemia on bloods and a mild elevation in urea consistent with chronic gastro-intestinal bleeding.

Question A
Select the ONE prescription that is most likely to be a cause of her black stools. Mark with a tick in column A.

Question B
Select the THREE prescriptions that are most likely to interact to cause her dry eyes. Mark with a tick in column B.

CURRENT PRESCRIPTIONS					
Drug name	Dose	Route	Freq.	A	B
Amitriptyline	75 mg	Oral	Daily	☐	☐
Aspirin	75 mg	Oral	Daily	☐	☐
Atorvastatin	40 mg	Oral	Daily	☐	☐
Bisoprolol	5 mg	Oral	Daily	☐	☐
Codeine phosphate	30 mg	Oral	6-hrly PRN	☐	☐
Chlorphenamine	4 mg	Oral	8-hrly PRN	☐	☐
Fultium® D3 (colecalciferol)	800 units	Oral	Daily	☐	☐
Glyceryl trinitrate 400 microgram spray	1–2 sprays	Oral	As required	☐	☐
Paracetamol	1 g	Oral	6-hrly PRN	☐	☐
Ramipril	5 mg	Oral	Daily	☐	☐

PLANNING MANAGEMENT (8 QUESTIONS, 2 MARKS EACH)

Q1. A 70-year-old man presents to the emergency department complaining of left-sided chest pain which is worse on breathing in deeply. He has just returned from a holiday to Thailand (during which he was well) a week ago but since his return has been troubled by a pain in his right leg. PMH: He has a PMH of systemic lupus and lupus nephritis which has led to chronic kidney disease. DH: He takes regular hydroxychloroquine and ramipril. He has no known drug allergies.

On examination

Temperature 36.5°C, HR 120/min and regular, BP 148/70 mmHg, JVP not raised, RR 30/min, O_2 sat 92% on 10 L/min, HS no murmur, chest auscultation is unremarkable.

Investigations

Na^+ 141 mmol/L (137–144), K^+ 4.9 mmol/L (3.5–4.9), urea 20 mmol/L (2.5–7.0), Cr 180 micromol/L (60–110), eGFR 25 mL/min/1.73m^2 (24 a month previously) [>60]
ECG shows sinus tachycardia.
CXR clear.

Question

Select the most appropriate management option at this stage. Mark with a tick.

MANAGEMENT OPTIONS		
A	Alteplase	☐
B	Aspirin	☐
C	Dabigatran	☐
D	Dalteparin	☐
E	Unfractionated heparin	☐

Q2. An 81-year-old man presents to the emergency department following a fall in the road. He notes that he has experienced episodes of feeling faint over the previous 4 weeks. PMH: He has previously been diagnosed with hypertension and gout and had a stroke in the past. He normally takes amlodipine, allopurinol and aspirin. SH: He lives on his own, is fully independent of activities of daily living and mobilizes with a walking stick.

On examination
HR 140/min and regular, BP 103/72 mmHg, JVP not raised, RR 12/min, O_2 sat 98% on air, HS normal, chest sounds vesicular with no added sounds. He is fully orientated and his AMTS is 10/10.

Investigations
ECG shows atrial fibrillation with a narrow QRS and ventricular rate of 120–140/min.
Electrolytes and thyroid function tests are normal.

Question
Select the most appropriate management option at this stage. Mark with a tick.

MANAGEMENT OPTIONS		
A	DC cardioversion	☐
B	Defibrillation	☐
C	Intravenous amiodarone	☐
D	Oral flecainide	☐
E	Oral metoprolol	☐

Q3. A 72-year-old woman presents to her GP surgery for her medication review. PMH: She has suffered from anxiety, depression and insomnia for over 20 years. DH: She has only taken temazepam at night for the last 5 years. SH: She was widowed 20 years ago and lives alone. She has two children who emigrated to Australia and Canada, respectively, 18 years ago.

Question
Select the most appropriate management option at this stage. Mark with a tick.

MANAGEMENT OPTIONS		
A	Stop the temazepam at an agreed stop date	☐
B	Switch to zopiclone as it has a safer side effect profile	☐
C	Switch to 5 mg diazepam and initiate a reduction programme of 1–2 mg fortnightly	☐
D	Continue this medication to manage this patient's long-term condition	☐
E	Stop the temazepam and commence an antidepressant in its place	☐

Q4. A 15-year-old boy (weighing 50 kg) presents via ambulance to paediatric HDU with severe breathlessness and difficulty breathing which has not responded adequately to his salbutamol inhaler. He has had high-flow oxygen en route via the ambulance. PMH: Asthma, perennial hay fever, and sensitivities to numerous household and environmental allergens. DH: He normally takes cetirizine, Clenil® Modulite 100 microgram inhaler, montelukast, prednisolone, salbutamol 100 microgram inhaler and Uniphyllin® Continus. SH: Non-smoker; lives with family.

On examination

Temperature 37.2°C, pulse 130/min and regular, BP 120/80 mmHg, RR 32/min, O_2 sat 90% on air, chest sounds suggest a widespread expiratory wheeze, and the child is unable to speak in sentences.

Investigations

CXR shows no significant findings except hyper-expansion of the lungs.

Question

Select the most appropriate management option at this stage. Mark with a tick.

	MANAGEMENT OPTIONS	
A	Aminophylline IV injection – 250 mg STAT	☐
B	Hydrocortisone IV injection – 100 mg STAT	☐
C	Ipratropium nebulised – 500 micrograms STAT	☐
D	Prednisolone tablets – 40 mg STAT dose	☐
E	Salbutamol 5 mg nebulised – 5 mg STAT	☐

Q5. A 6-year-old child (weighing 25 kg) presents to the paediatric assessment unit with a 3-day history of fever, vomiting and diarrhoea. PMH: Nil. DH: Nil. SH: Lives with family.

On examination

Sunken eyes, dry lips, temperature 38.8°C, pulse 120/min and regular, BP 110/60 mmHg, RR 25/min, O_2 sat 98% on air, and CRT 3 sec.

Investigations

Na^+ 130 mmol/L (137–144), K^+ 5.2 mmol/L (3.5–4.9), urea 8.1 mmol/L (2.5–7.0), Cr 115 micromol/L (60–110), eGFR 25 mL/min/1.73 m² (<60)

Question

Select the most appropriate fluid management option at this stage. Mark with a tick.

	MANAGEMENT OPTIONS	
A	Give replacement intravenous fluid using 0.45% sodium chloride at two-thirds maintenance	☐
B	Give replacement intravenous fluid using 0.18% sodium chloride with 4% glucose and 20 mmol potassium	☐
C	Give an intravenous bolus of 10 mL/kg of glucose 10% to help correct intravascular depletion	☐
D	Give an intravenous bolus of 10–20 mL/kg of 0.9% sodium chloride to correct for intravascular depletion	☐
E	Give an oral rehydration sachet mixed with 200 mL of water to the child as needed	☐

Q6. A 24-year-old woman presents to the Emergency Pregnancy Assessment Unit (EPAU) complaining of heavy PV bleeding and pain in the back and abdomen region. She is believed to be 10 weeks pregnant. PMH: G4P2. DH: Nil regular.

Investigations
A TA/TV USS shows a single IU pregnancy and no foetal heart pulsations are seen. Both ovaries are normal in appearance, no mass is seen and the right endometrium is thickened.

Question
Select the most appropriate management option for the miscarriage at this stage for this woman. Mark with a tick.

MANAGEMENT OPTIONS	
A	Medical management using mifepristone
B	Surgical management to remove POC
C	Conservative management with pain relief and support advice
D	Re-book for a second TA/TV scan
E	Discharge home with advice to return to ED if the problem persists or worsens

Q7. A 32-year-old woman of Asian origin presents to the emergency department complaining of redness and itching across her body, especially on the palms of her hand and soles of her feet, for the past two weeks. She is known to be 27 weeks pregnant. PMH: Nil. DH: Nil.

On examination

Upon skin inspection you note no visible rash or signs suggestive of eczema. Upon questioning the woman tells you she has also noticed darker urine recently.

Investigations

Na$^+$ 142 mmol/L (137–144), K$^+$ 4.3 mmol/L (3.5–4.9), urea 6.0 mmol/L (2.5 – 7.0), Cr 71 micromol/L (60–110), ALT 129 U/L (5–35), AST 127 U/L (1–31), ALP 127 U/L (45–105), PT – 13.5 sec (11.5–16.5)

Question

Select the most appropriate management option for the condition this woman has presented with. Mark with a tick.

MANAGEMENT OPTIONS		
A	Undertake a viral screen for hepatitis A–C, EBV and CMV	☐
B	Refer this patient back to her GP for GP-led care	☐
C	Offer this women the option of an early elective delivery	☐
D	Prescribe a topical anti-pruritic emollient to help with the pruritus short term	☐
E	Prescribe ursodeoxycholic acid to improve pruritus and liver function	☐

Q8. An 82-year-old man is brought to the emergency department having been found next to an empty packet of amitriptyline. He is now complaining of blurred vision. PMH: He has suffered from depression, hypertension and ischaemic heart disease. DH: He normally takes amitriptyline, aspirin, bisoprolol and ramipril. SH: He lives alone and is recently bereaved.

On examination
Temperature 36.9°C, HR 90/min and regular, BP 110/75 mmHg.

Investigations
Cardiac monitor and ECG show runs of non-sustained ventricular tachycardia.

Question
Select the most appropriate management option at this stage. Mark with a tick.

MANAGEMENT OPTIONS		
A	Active monitoring	☐
B	Amiodarone infusion	☐
C	DC cardioversion	☐
D	Magnesium sulphate infusion	☐
E	Sodium bicarbonate infusion	☐

COMMUNICATING INFORMATION (6 QUESTIONS, 2 MARKS EACH)

Q1. A 28-year-old woman presents to her GP surgery asking for pre-conception advice. PMH: She has suffered from petit mal epilepsy. DH: She normally takes levetiracetam. SH: She lives with her partner and she is a deputy bank manager.

Question

Select the most appropriate information option that should be communicated to the patient. Mark with a tick.

	INFORMATION OPTIONS	
A	She should be advised that she needs folic acid supplementation	☐
B	She should be encouraged to notify the UK Epilepsy and Pregnancy Register	☐
C	She should be referred to a specialist to be given further pre-conception advice	☐
D	She should be advised to switch to sodium valproate	☐
E	She should be advised to stop her medications with immediate effect	☐

Q2. A 62-year-old woman presents to her GP with a prescription request from her recent eye clinic appointment for latanoprost. PMH: She has just been diagnosed with open angle glaucoma in her left eye. DH: Nil. SH: She lives alone.

Question

Select the most appropriate information option that should be communicated to the patient. Mark with a tick.

	INFORMATION OPTIONS	
A	Latanoprost drops should be instilled in the evening	☐
B	Latanoprost can darken the pigment of the iris	☐
C	Latanoprost should be used with caution in asthma	☐
D	Latanoprost can cause headaches	☐
E	Latanoprost should be used in caution with high blood pressure	☐

Q3. A 10-month-old child is brought to the GP by her mum who is complaining of the child having a 'gunky' red eye. The child has had symptoms of an URTI for the past few days. The red eye was apparent since the morning of the presentation and the child has not been noted to have any previous mucoid discharge in the eyes. **PMH:** The child is up to date with his immunizations. **DH:** Nil. **Allergies:** Nil. **SH:** The parents are in a stable relationship.

Question

Select the most appropriate information option that should be communicated to the mother. Mark with a tick.

	INFORMATION OPTIONS	
A	The child should be started on topical chloramphenicol treatment	☐
B	The child should be started on topical fusidic acid drops	☐
C	A swab should be taken and results awaited before starting any treatment	☐
D	The mother should be reassured that the lacrimal duct is immature and so discharge is likely to be due to this	☐
E	The mother should be advised to have a vaginal swab for chlamydia and gonorrhoea	☐

Q4. A 12-month-old child presents to your GP surgery with his mother for his routine childhood immunizations. **PMH:** Nil. **DH:** Nil. **SH:** Lives with parents and has no siblings.

Question

Select the most appropriate information option that should be communicated to the mother. Mark with a tick.

	INFORMATION OPTIONS	
A	The child will only be having two vaccinations today	☐
B	This child will be having two booster vaccines	☐
C	The MMR vaccine is not safe for this child	☐
D	If the child is ill with 'cold-like symptoms' close to the appointment, he will not be able to have the MMR vaccine	☐
E	The mum can collect the vaccines using the FP10 they are to be issued prior to the appointment	☐

Q5. A 54-year-old woman presents to the gynaecology assessment unit (GAU) complaining of bouts of abdominal cramping pain with suprapubic tenderness and an associated loss of appetite. Upon investigation she is diagnosed as having PID. PMH: Oophorectomy 7 years ago; post-menopausal. No history of previous STIs. DH: She has been started on co-codamol, doxycycline and metronidazole.

Question

Select the most appropriate information option that should be communicated to the patient about her treatment with metronidazole tablets. Mark with a tick.

	INFORMATION OPTIONS	
A	She must avoid alcohol containing products	☐
B	She should stop taking the tablets once she is feeling better	☐
C	She should take the tablets on an empty stomach	☐
D	She can crush or chew the tablets	☐
E	She must take the tablets with small amounts of water	☐

Q6. An 18-year-old single mother presents to her GP surgery complaining of depression. You take a history and elicit a PHQ 9 score of 19. She reports not having any intention of suicide. PMH: Chlamydia. PSH: 2x TOP, laparoscopy for division of adhesions. DH: Nil. SH: **She has a 3-year-old child, and her mother suffers from alcoholism.**

You decide that she needs to be started on an SSRI and opt for fluoxetine.

Question

Select the most appropriate information option that should be communicated to the patient.

	INFORMATION OPTIONS	
A	This drug can sometimes cause a rash	☐
B	Should she suffer from suicidal intention in the first 2 weeks of initiation, this will result in immediate withdrawal of the drug	☐
C	Cheese and wine should be avoided concomitantly due to a possible dietary tyramine induced hypertensive crisis	☐
D	The drug should not be taken at same time as a tricyclic antidepressant due to serotonin syndrome	☐
E	This drug can sometimes cause a loss of libido	☐

CALCULATION SKILLS (8 QUESTIONS, 2 MARKS EACH)

Q1. A 20-year-old man presents to the accident and emergency department complaining of chest pain. This is found to be due to a pneumothorax that requires aspiration which is unfortunately unsuccessful. He therefore requires insertion of a chest drain. He has already received 5 mL of 2% lidocaine subcutaneously as anaesthesia for the aspiration 20 minutes earlier. He weighs 70 kg.

The maximum dose of lidocaine is 3 mg/kg.

Calculation

What is the remaining volume of 2% lidocaine that may be used subcutaneously during the chest drain insertion? Write your answer in the box below.

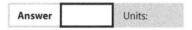

Q2. An 81-year-old woman presents to the acute medical unit complaining of abdominal pain. She was diagnosed a year ago with metastatic colorectal carcinoma and is now on fully palliative treatment. The pain is so severe that she is currently taking as required oral morphine sulphate 15 mg every hour, on top of a fentanyl patch (75 micrograms/hour) together with laxative and anti-emetic cover. The decision is made to deliver current analgesia via a subcutaneous constant infusion of diamorphine as she is imminently dying.

Calculation

Using the conversions below, calculate how many milligrams of diamorphine should be included in a 24-hour subcutaneous infusion.

Fentanyl 75 micrograms/hour patch	≡ 300 mg oral morphine sulphate in 24 hours
Diamorphine 10 mg	≡ 30 mg oral morphine sulphate in 24 hours

Write your answer in the box below.

Answer [ ] Units:

Q3. A 27-year-old man with hypoparathyroidism who usually takes a 2 microgram dose of alfacalcidol oral drops is admitted to an acute medical ward. You are required to prescribe this medication on his electronic prescribing chart.

Calculation

How many drops of alfacalcidol should you prescribe? Write your answer in the box below.

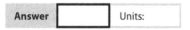

Q4. A 27-year-old man presents to your GP surgery with symptoms suggestive of an acute flare-up of his eczema. You are required to prescribe Betnovate-RD® ointment for a 2-week application to both of his hands and arms, as well as his trunk.

Calculation
How many 100 g tubes should you prescribe? Write your answer in the box below.

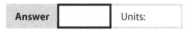

Q5. A 43-year-old man weighing 145 kg is due for bariatric surgery. You are required to calculate the current body surface area (BSA) for this patient as this will be important when dosing drugs.

Calculation
Given that the patient is 160 cm tall, calculate his current BSA using the following equation:

$$\text{BSA}\left(\text{m}^2\right) = \sqrt{\left(\text{height (cm)} \times \text{weight (kg)} / 3600\right)}.$$

Write your answer in the box below.

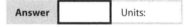

Q6. A 29-year-old women presents to the GAU for repeat bloods and beta-HCG prior to receiving subcutaneous methotrexate for her ectopic pregnancy. Beta-HCG returns at 2560, and all other pathological results are normal.

The dose specified in your local guidelines is 50 mg/m² (up to a maximum of 100 mg). The patient weighs 80 kg and is 1.56 m tall.

Calculation
What total dose should the patient receive? Write your answer in the box below.

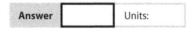

Q7. A 5-year-old child has been brought to the surgery by her mum with symptoms of a UTI with a temperature of 37.8°C. An MSU sample which you dipstick is positive for nitrites and leucocytes. She has no symptoms of ascending infection. You consult the local antimicrobial guidelines and decide to prescribe trimethoprim 50 mg/5 mL suspension. Your weighing scales are broken and the mum doesn't know the weight of the child.

Calculation

Given that a child's weight can be estimated by the formula (age + 4) × 2 and that trimethoprim is prescribed at a dose of 4 mg/kg (max. 200 mg) every 12 hours in a child aged 1 month–12 years, at what dose should the trimethoprim be prescribed? Write your answer in the box below.

Answer		Units:

Q8. A 2-day-old child presents to the paediatric emergency department with his parents who are complaining of the child having recurrent seizures. You are required to give a dose of midazolam as an IV injection initially at a suitable dose. The patient weighs 3.5 kg.

Calculation

What dose should the patient be given? Write your answer in the box below.

Answer		Units:

ADVERSE DRUG REACTIONS (8 QUESTIONS, 2 MARKS EACH)

Q1. A 14-year-old boy presents to hospital with suspected cellulitis secondary to a rugby injury one week ago. Following an aspirate and blood cultures he is started on intravenous gentamicin and flucloxacillin. This fails to help the condition, and microbiology advise stopping the flucloxacillin and adding in clindamycin. PMH: Asthma. DH: Beclamethasone 100 microgram inhaler and salbutamol 100 microgram inhaler.

Question type A
Select the adverse effect that is most likely to be caused by clindamycin. Mark with a tick.

PRESCRIPTION OPTIONS		
A	Acute kidney injury	☐
B	Diarrhoea	☐
C	Electrolyte disturbances	☐
D	Ototoxicity	☐
E	Rash	☐

Q2. A 46-year-old woman is reviewed in a menopause clinic and is started on Evorel® Conti '50' patches to help control symptoms of the climacteric. PMH: Hypothyroidism. DH: Levothyroxine.

Question type A
Select the adverse effect that is most likely to be caused by this treatment. Mark with a tick.

PRESCRIPTION OPTIONS		
A	Abdominal cramps	☐
B	Breast cancer	☐
C	Endometrial cancer	☐
D	Ovarian cancer	☐
E	Venous thromboembolism	☐

Q3. An 85-year-old woman is referred into the acute medical unit by her GP after an incidental finding of a potassium of 6.5 mmol/L (3.5–4.9). She has a history of ischaemic cardiomyopathy, having had two previous myocardial infarctions and was recently treated for a urinary tract infection. She normally takes aspirin, clopidogrel, atorvastatin, candesartan, metoprolol, epleronone and furosemide and is on day 2 of a course of trimethoprim.

Question type B
Select the prescription that is most likely to be contributing to this patient's hyperkalaemia. Mark with a tick.

PRESCRIPTION OPTIONS		
A	Aspirin	☐
B	Atorvastatin	☐
C	Candesartan	☐
D	Clopidogrel	☐
E	Eplerenone	☐
F	Furosemide	☐
G	Metoprolol	☐
H	Trimethoprim	☐

Q4. A 59-year-old woman presents to her GP complaining of a rash. PMH: Hypothyroidism, type 2 diabetes, CKD3 and bipolar disorder. DH: She normally takes gliclazide, lithium, levothyroxine, metformin and ramipril. SH: None.

On examination
The rash is salmon-pink coloured in well-demarcated plaques, with a scaly texture, and is on her scalp predominantly but also on her extensor surfaces.

Question type B
Select the prescription that is most likely to be contributing to the rash. Mark with a tick.

PRESCRIPTION OPTIONS		
A	Gliclazide	☐
B	Levothyroxine	☐
C	Lithium	☐
D	Metformin	☐
E	Ramipril	☐

Q5. A 29-year-old African-Caribbean man presents to his GP surgery complaining of constipation. PMH: He has suffered from schizophrenia since 22 years of age and has a history of chronic back pain. DH: He normally takes zopiclone, mirtazapine, clozapine, omeprazole, paracetamol, codeine phosphate and beclomethasone nasal spray. SH: He smokes three joints of cannabis daily.

Question type C
Select the prescription that is most likely to have interacted with codeine phosphate to cause constipation. Mark with a tick.

PRESCRIPTION OPTIONS		
A	Beclomethasone	☐
B	Clozapine	☐
C	Mirtazapine	☐
D	Omeprazole	☐
E	Zopiclone	☐

Q6. A 54-year-old obese woman presents to her GP complaining of agitation, extreme anxiety and insomnia. She was started on citalopram 1 month ago for depression. PMH: Hypothyroidism, OA left ankle, type 2 diabetes and CKD3. PSH: Bimalleolar fracture left ankle 5 years ago. DH: She normally takes gliclazide, levothyroxine, metformin, ramipril and tramadol. SH: Widow for the past 2 years.

Question type C
Select the prescription that is most likely to interact with citalopram to cause her symptoms. Mark with a tick.

PRESCRIPTION OPTIONS		
A	Gliclazide	☐
B	Levothyroxine	☐
C	Metformin	☐
D	Ramipril	☐
E	Tramadol M/R	☐

Q7. An 83-year-old man has developed a severe blistering rash after commencing naproxen for osteoarthritis of the knees. He is diagnosed with toxic epidermal necrolysis and admitted to the intensive care unit.

Question type D

Select the management option that is most appropriate for the rash. Mark with a tick.

	PRESCRIPTION OPTIONS	
A	Cooling measures	☐
B	Dermovate® ointment	☐
C	Debridement of blisters	☐
D	Oral prednisolone	☐
E	Stop naproxen	☐

Q8. A 19-year-old woman who is being treated on your obstetrics and gynaecology ward is noticed by a nurse as having facial grimacing and lip-smacking. PMH: She has been in three times in the last 6 weeks for severe hyperemesis. DH: She is currently on cyclizine, metoclopramide, multivitamin tablets, ondansetron and thiamine.

Question type D

Select the management that is most appropriate for the facial twitching. Mark with a tick.

	PRESCRIPTION OPTIONS	
A	Procyclidine	☐
B	Benztropine (IV)	☐
C	Carbamazepine (PO)	☐
D	Magnesium sulphate (IV)	☐
E	Methyldopa (PO)	☐

DRUG MONITORING (8 QUESTIONS, 2 MARKS EACH)

Q1. A 38-year-old woman presents to the endocrine clinic with a history of type 1 diabetes, complicated by diabetic nephropathy. She states that her blood sugars have been erratic of late. DH: She normally takes 15 units of Novomix-30® in the morning and evening, as well as ramipril.

Question
Select the most important monitoring option to assess her insulin dosing. Mark with a tick.

MONITORING OPTIONS		
A	Urine dipstick	☐
B	HbA$_{1c}$ levels	☐
C	Number of hypoglycaemic episodes	☐
D	Lipid profile	☐
E	Blood pressure	☐

Q2. A 54-year-old woman presents to the rheumatology clinic complaining of a 4-week history of joint pain affecting her hands and knees which had commenced soon after an episode of diarrhoea. PMH: She has no medical history. DH: She has been taking Voltarol® gel for the pain. SH: She is a violin teacher and lives with her husband and two children.

On examination she has tender, swollen metacarpophalyngeal joints and knees. A reducing dose of steroids are commenced on this admission, commencing at 20 mg prednisolone.

Question
Select the most appropriate monitoring option when you see her in 6 weeks to assess the beneficial effects of this treatment. Mark with a tick.

MONITORING OPTIONS		
A	Repeat radiographs for development of inflammatory changes	☐
B	Serial C-reactive protein	☐
C	Serial erythrocyte sedimentation rate	☐
D	Disease Activity Score (DAS28)	☐
E	Clinical monitoring	☐

Q3. A 23-year-old woman presents to the infectious diseases clinic for an HIV review. PMH: She was diagnosed with HIV 5 years previously when she presented with oesophageal candida. DH: She normally takes an anti-retroviral regime which includes tenofovir.

She is well and is due to be reviewed again in 6 months' time.

Question
Which of the following would be most appropriately monitored on a 3–6 monthly basis? Mark with a tick.

MONITORING OPTIONS		
A	Cardiovascular disease risk	☐
B	CD4 cell count	☐
C	Cervical cytology	☐
D	HbA$_{1c}$	☐
E	Urinalysis	☐

Q4. A 56-year-old African-Caribbean man presents to his GP for a medication review following blood tests in preparation for the review. The total cholesterol on the blood tests was 5.3 mmol/L. He has never been tried on a statin. PMH: He had an MI 5 years ago. DH: Nil. SH: He smokes 20/day.

On examination
BP 139/83, BMI 32.

You decide to start him on simvastatin 40 mg.

Question
Select the most appropriate monitoring option to assess the adverse effects of this treatment. Mark with a tick.

MONITORING OPTIONS		
A	Baseline CK and annually thereafter	☐
B	Baseline CK and repeated if any symptoms of muscle pains thereafter	☐
C	LFTs at 12 months	☐
D	Annual LFTs and CK	☐
E	Baseline LFT and CK, repeat LFT after 3 and 12 months of initiation of simvastatin and CK if muscle pains thereafter	☐

Q5. An 81-year-old woman is brought to A&E by ambulance with symptoms of acute wheeziness and shortness of breath. PMH: Asthma, alcohol dependence and CCF. DH: Beclomethasone inhaler, bisoprolol, bumetanide and ramipril. SH: She is a non-smoker.

She has been commenced on nebulizers but to little effect and is started on an aminophylline infusion for an acute severe asthma attack.

Question
Select the most appropriate monitoring option to assess the adverse effects of this treatment. Mark with a tick.

MONITORING OPTIONS		
A	Bedside cardiac monitoring	☐
B	Theophylline levels at 4–6 hours	☐
C	Serial spirometry every hour	☐
D	Aminophylline levels at 4–6 hours	☐
E	Theophylline levels after 12 hours	☐

Q6. A 52-year-old man presents to the CMHT for his annual mental health review. He is complaining of weight gain. PMH: He has suffered from schizophrenia for 20 years. DH: He normally takes quetiapine. SH: He lives alone in social housing on long-term incapacity benefits.

Question
Select the most appropriate monitoring option to assess the adverse effects of this treatment. Mark with a tick.

MONITORING OPTIONS		
A	Annual ECG	☐
B	Annual fasting lipids and glucose	☐
C	6-monthly height and weight	☐
D	Annual FBC and fasting lipids and glucose	☐
E	Annual BMI, fasting lipids and glucose, FBC and ECG	☐

Q7. A 12-year-old boy is admitted on to paediatric HDU with diabetic ketoacidosis. PMH: Type 1 diabetic. DH: Lantus Solostar® Pen and NovoRapid FlexPen®. SH: Nil.

Question

Select the most appropriate initial monitoring option to assess whether the child has diabetic ketoacidosis. Mark with a tick.

	MONITORING OPTIONS	
A	Arterial blood gases	☐
B	Serum calcium level	☐
C	Serum potassium level	☐
D	Blood glucose level	☐
E	Blood culture	☐

Q8. A 33-year-old woman who is prescribed methotrexate by you under a shared care agreement for an inflammatory joint disorder presents to your surgery for a routine appointment for her 3-monthly monitoring.

Question

Select the most appropriate monitoring option to assess the beneficial effect of this treatment. Mark with a tick.

	MONITORING OPTIONS	
A	Erythrocyte sedimentation rate	☐
B	Full blood counts	☐
C	Liver function tests	☐
D	Pro-collagen 3 protein	☐
E	Urea and electrolytes	☐

DATA INTERPRETATION (6 QUESTIONS, 2 MARKS EACH)

Q1. A 20-year-old man presents to the GUM clinic complaining of dysuria. PMH: He has suffered from asthma, requiring three previous hospitalizations, and is severely atopic with a history of anaphylaxis to penicillin and peanuts. DH: He uses a budesonide inhaler, monteleukast and PRN salbutamol to control his asthma. SH: He is a non-smoker who drinks 16 units a week and has recently returned from a holiday in Majorca.

Urinalysis reveals

Protein	+
Blood	+
Leukocytes	++++
Glucose	−
Ketones	−

Microscopy reveals gram-negative diplococci.

Question

Select the most appropriate decision option with regard to the next management step based on these data. Mark with a tick.

DECISION OPTIONS		
A	Prescribe a course of oral doxycycline empirically	☐
B	Prescribe a course oral co-amoxiclav empirically	☐
C	Await culture sensitivities to reduce the risk of treatment failure	☐
D	Prescribe a single intramuscular dose of cefalexin	☐
E	Perform dark ground microscopy prior to commencing therapy	☐

Q2. An 83-year-old woman is admitted to the neuro-rehab unit following a total anterior circulation stroke with residual aphasia and cognitive deficit. She has become increasingly confused and her oral intake has reduced. Ten days previously she completed a 3-day course of nitrofurantoin for a positive urine dip. PMH: She has suffered from hypercholesterolaemia, constipation and transient ischaemic attacks previously. DH: She normally takes atorvastatin, aspirin, clopidogrel and movicol. She has a penicillin allergy.

Examination
She is febrile at 38.0, heart rate is 110 and BP 130/93, RR 17, sat 99% (on air). She is hot to touch and tender in the right upper quadrant.

Investigations
CRP 256 (<15), ALT 454 U/L (5–35), WCC 16 × 10⁹/L (4–11), ALP 42 U/L (45–105), urea 9.1 mmol/L (2.5–7.0), GGT 450 U/L (4–35), Cr 70 micromol/L (60–110), bilirubin 17 micromol/L (1–22)
Urine normal.
CXR normal.
Ultrasound abdomen: Dilated common bile duct and inflammatory change within the wall of the gall bladder

Question
Select the most appropriate decision option with regard to the management of this patient's sepsis based on these data. Mark with a tick.

DECISION OPTIONS	
A	Co-amoxiclav (IV)	☐
B	Ciprofloxacin (PO), gentamicin (IV) and metronidazole (PO)	☐
C	Ceftriaxone (IV) and metronidazole (IV)	☐
D	Trimethoprim (PO)	☐
E	Ciprofloxacin (IV), gentamicin (IV) and fluconazole (IV)	☐

Q3. An 83-year-old woman presents to the emergency department complaining of a history of brown diarrhoea and vomiting. PMH: She has hypertension and vitamin D deficiency. DH: She normally takes amlodipine and colecalciferol. SH: She is independent and lives in sheltered accommodation.

Examination
Her JVP is not visible and she has dry oral mucosa. Her blood pressure is 100/65 mmHg.

Investigations
Arterial blood gas: FiO$_2$ 21%, pH 7.53 (7.35–7.45), pO$_2$ 13.0 kPa (11.3–12.6), pCO$_2$ 4.5 kPa (4.7–6.0), HCO$_3$ 24.1 mmol/L (21–29), lactate 1.9 mmol/L (0.5–1.6), base excess 4.3 (−2 to +2)
Bloods: Na$^+$ 134 mmol/L (137–144), K$^+$ 2.1 mmol/L (3.5–4.9), Cl$^-$ 90 mmol/L (95–107), urea 8.1 mmol/L (2.5–7.0), Cr 86 micromol/L (60–110).
ECG: Sinus rhythm with a rate of 60, narrow QRS complexes and flattening of the T waves throughout.

Question
Select the most appropriate decision option with regard to the management of her hypokalaemia based on these data. Mark with a tick.

	DECISION OPTIONS	
A	500 mL of 0.9% sodium chloride containing 40 mmol potassium	☐
B	500 mL of 5% glucose containing 40 mmol potassium	☐
C	1 L of 0.9% sodium chloride containing 40 mmol potassium	☐
D	1 L of 5% glucose containing 40 mmol potassium	☐
E	1 L of Hartmann's solution	☐

Q4. A 56-year-old woman presents to the A&E via an ambulance complaining of dyspnoea. PMH: She has suffered from chronic obstructive pulmonary disease. DH: She normally takes Seretide® 500 accuhaler, theophylline and azithromycin and has regular home nebulized ipratropium and salbutamol and home oxygen (0.5 L/min).

Examination
Temperature 36.9°C, HR 95 bpm, BP 110/82, RR 15, sat 87% on 5 L/min, GCS 15/15.

Chest auscultation reveals widespread wheeze.

Investigations
Arterial blood gas: pH 7.32 (7.35–7.45), PaO$_2$ 18.1 kPa (10.0–14.0), PaCO$_2$ 8.5 kPa (4.4–5.9), bicarbonate 29 mmol/L (22–26)

Question
Select the most appropriate decision option with regard to the management of this patient based on these data. Mark with a tick.

DECISION OPTIONS		
A	BiPAP	☐
B	CPAP	☐
C	Oxygen 2 L/min via nasal specula	☐
D	Oxygen 28% via Venturi mask	☐
E	Oxygen 35% via Venturi mask	☐

Q5. A 36-year-old woman presents to her GP surgery complaining of tension headaches. She has been followed up for the past 3 months. PMH: She has suffered from IBS, ovarian cyst and mild depression. DH: She normally takes Fybogel®, mebeverine, citalopram and Microgynon® 30 for contraception. SH: Non-smoker.

On examination

BMI: 31 kg/m².

In the preceding 3 months, her last 3 BP readings have been 146/93, 153/89 and 148/99 mmHg.

Question

Select the most appropriate decision option with regard to the Microgynon 30 prescription based on these data. Mark with a tick.

DECISION OPTIONS		
A	Immediately stop all types of hormonal contraception	☐
B	Immediately stop Microgynon 30	☐
C	Continue Microgynon 30 until end of pack then switch to a progesterone-only pill	☐
D	Continue on Microgynon 30 but advise that the patient loses some weight	☐
E	Continue Microgynon 30 until end of pack then switch to contraceptive patch	☐

Q6. An 18-year-old woman is brought to A&E by ambulance having taken 12 paracetamol tablets 7 hours ago, deliberately. PMH: Anorexia nervosa. DH: Nil. SH: Parents separated 12 months ago. Sibling died in an RTA 3 months ago.

On examination
GCS 15/15, BP 113/72 mmHg, pulse 88, weight 36 kg.

Investigations
INR 1.0 (0.8–1.2), urea 4.5 mmol/L (135–145), Cr 76 micromol/L (60–110), ALT 42 U/L (0–45), PaO_2 12 (10.0–14.0 kPa), $PaCO_2$ 5.1 (4.4–5.9 kPa), bicarbonate 22 mmol/L (22–26)
Blood tests show a blood paracetamol level of 65 mg/L.

Question
Select the most appropriate decision option with regard to the treatment of the overdose based on these data. Mark with a tick.

DECISION OPTIONS		
A	Wait for 8 hours post overdose then start N-acetylcysteine due to the delayed gastric emptying effect	☐
B	Administer activated charcoal immediately and commence gastric lavage	☐
C	Start N-acetylcysteine as soon as possible, regardless of the blood concentration level	☐
D	Start N-acetylcysteine as soon as the blood concentration levels are obtained	☐
E	Admit and monitor blood and clinical indices for 24 hours and take advice from Toxbase/ NPIS	☐

PSA Paper One – Answers and Rationale

PRESCRIBING

Q1

- This child has presented with reflux (GORD). This is not routinely treated unless two or more of the following are present:
  - Disturbed feeding pattern (poor feeding, refusal of food, choking and regurgitation)
  - Distressed behaviour (irritable behaviour and crying)
  - Lack of growth (poor weight gain and faltering growth)
  - An episode of pneumonia
  - Chronic cough
  - Hoarse voice
- In this instance a breastfeeding assessment has been carried out and the symptoms have still persisted. Thus it is important to start an alginate for an initial 1–2 week trial.
- The use of a proton pump inhibitor or H2-receptor antagonist is not indicated initially and there may be licensing implications especially in children.
- Domperidone is no longer routinely indicated for reflux due to recent MHRA advice surrounding cardiac concerns; however, it may be used in certain situations. For more information around this, please review Ref. (3).
- If the mother was bottle feeding, we may want to use a different stepped-care approach which does not involve an alginate at first. For example, we may want to reduce feed volumes, give smaller more frequent feeds, use a thickened formula and so on.
- For more details on this topic, review Ref. (4).

The correct answer is:

Mark(s)	Criteria			Answer		
4	Optimal drug choice			Gaviscon® Infant Sachets		
4	Dosage	Route	Frequency	1 dose	Oral (mixed with water)	Max 6 × daily
1	Timing			PRN		
1	Signature			Signature		

- Previously Gaviscon Infant Sachets were prescribed as either 'half-a-dual-sachet' or 'one-sachet'. However, it is now recommended to pre-scribe as 'one dose' (for those <4.5 kg) or 'two doses' (for those >4.5 kg), respectively.

Q2

- This patient has moderate hypertension and the drug of choice should be labetalol at an initial dose of 100 mg BD, which can be titrated up to 200 mg BD or greater based on clinical response.
- Other potential agents include suitable beta adreno-receptor blockers, nifedipine and methyldopa.
- For more information on hypertension in pregnancy, please refer to NICE clinical guidance 107 – *Hypertension in Pregnancy* (January 2011) (5).
- In this patient, it is also important to rule out HELLP syndrome (hae-molysis, elevated liver enzymes and low platelet count). Pathological markers seem fine on this occasion, but if they were not we would need to consider a diagnosis of (pre)-eclampsia which usually pres-ents with neurological problems (headaches and visual disturbances), as well as abdominal pain, swelling (hands, feet and/or face) and vomiting.
- For more information on the above point, please refer to NICE Clinical Guidance 62 – *Antenatal Care* (6).

The correct answer is:

Mark(s)	Criteria			Answer		
4	Optimal drug choice			Labetalol		
4	Dosage	Route	Frequency	100 mg	Oral	BD
1	Timing			12 hours apart		
1	Signature			Signature		

Sub-optimal choices for which the drug choice mark will be reduced are:

- Another suitable beta adreno-receptor blocker (e.g. atenolol or meto-prolol) – 3 marks awarded out of 4.
- Nifedipine – 3 marks awarded out of 4.
- Hydralazine – 2 marks awarded out of 4.
- Methyldopa – 1 mark awarded out of 4 (due to risk of postnatal depression).
- ACEIs – 1 mark awarded out of 4 (certain ACEIs such as captopril and enalapril should be avoided especially in pre-term infants due to the risk of profound neonatal hypotension unless careful blood pressure monitoring occurs).
- Diuretic therapy (e.g. thiazide) – 0 marks awarded out of 4 (can lead to increased thirst in lactating mothers).

Q3

The correct answer is:

Mark(s)	Criteria			Answer		
4	Optimal drug choice			Adrenaline		
4	Dosage	Route	Frequency	300 micrograms	IM	STAT
1	Timing			Immediately		
1	Signature			Signature		

- This patient has an anaphylactic reaction to penicillin. Anaphylaxis is a medical emergency and it is vital that junior doctors know the correct dose of adrenaline to give.
- Chlorphenamine and steroids (usually in the form of hydrocortisone) are also given but are of secondary importance compared to adrenaline.

Sub-optimal choices for which the drug choice mark will be reduced are:

- Chlorphenamine 10 mg (IM or slow IV) – 1 mark awarded out of 4.
- Hydrocortisone 200 mg (IV) – 1 mark awarded out of 4.
- Fluid bolus – 1 mark awarded out of 4.

Q4

The correct answer is:

Mark(s)	Criteria			Answer		
4	Optimal drug choice			Beclomethasone 200 microgram inhaler		
4	Dosage	Route	Frequency	2 puffs	Inhaled	BD
1	Timing			Morning and evening		
1	Signature			Signature		

- This question is testing your knowledge of the BTS/SIGN guidance on the management of asthma in adults. The adjustments in therapy are based around five 'steps' and are worth being familiar with.
- In the case above the patient is uncontrolled despite the addition of a long-acting beta-agonist which has provided some benefit. Before the addition of other drugs, the recommendation is for inhaled corticosteroid to be increased to 800 micrograms/day.

Q5

The correct answer is:

Mark(s)	Criteria			Answer		
4	Optimal drug choice			Vancomycin		
4	Dosage	Route	Frequency	125 mg	Oral	QDS
1	Timing			6 hours apart (for 10–14 days)		
1	Signature			Signature		

- *Clostridium difficile* infection is an understandably hot topic nationally and politically as it is directly related to an iatrogenic cause.
- As soon as a *C. difficile* infection is considered:
  - Current antibiotic therapy should be re-assessed and discontinued if appropriate.
  - The severity of infection should be assessed.
- The following parameters indicate a severe infection requiring treatment with oral vancomycin rather than oral metronidazole (the treatment for non-severe infection):
  - Acute rise in creatinine.
  - Evidence of colitis (fresh red rectal bleeding or radiographic evidence on plain film or CT scan).
  - White cell count >15.

Q6

The correct answer is:

Mark(s)	Criteria			Answer		
4	Optimal drug choice			Amoxicillin		
4	Dosage	Route	Frequency	250 mg	Oral	TDS
1	Timing			8 hourly		
1	Signature			Signature		

- This child has signs of otitis media and the symptoms of disease have lasted longer than 72 hours. He also has signs of systemic illness as he has a reduced appetite and is irritable and also he has signs of complications with the mastoid tenderness. He therefore needs a course of antibiotics.

Sub-optimal choices for which the drug choice mark will be reduced are:

- Amoxil® – 3 marks awarded out of 4 (brand names should not be used routinely).
- Clarithromycin – 2 marks awarded out of 4 (only used in cases of penicillin allergy).
- Amoxicillin (intravenous or intramuscular) – 1 mark awarded out of 4 (oral route is first line).

Q7

The correct answers are:

Mark(s)	Criteria			Answer		
4	Optimal drug choice			Metoclopramide		
4	Dosage	Route	Frequency	10 mg	Oral	TDS
1	Timing			8 hourly		
1	Signature			Signature		

Mark(s)	Criteria			Answer		
4	Optimal drug choice			Ondansetron		
4	Dosage	Route	Frequency	4 or 8 mg	Oral	BD
1	Timing			12 hourly		
1	Signature			Signature		

- The treatment for nausea/vomiting depends on the severity. Most pregnancies at <8 weeks gestation are associated with nausea which normally resolves by 12 weeks.
- All anti-emetics are unlicensed in pregnancy.
- First-line treatment is PO cyclizine/PO promethazine and a favourable response should be seen in 24 hours. Second-line treatment is PO metoclopramide/PO ondansetron.
- Signs for admission include inability to tolerate fluids, postural hypotension, electrolyte imbalance and ketonuria (as a sign of starvation). Treatment should include IV fluids, PO/IV anti-emetic and vitamin B1 to avoid the complication of Wernicke's encephalopathy.

Sub-optimal choices for which the drug choice mark will be reduced are:

- Prochlorperazine – 2 marks awarded out of 4 (this is mentioned as second line in the BNF but is not in accordance with current NICE guidelines; it is known to cause extrapyramidal side effects and withdrawal in neonates if used in third-trimester pregnancy).
- Cyclizine – 1 mark awarded out of 4 (promethazine has already been tried, so trying an alternative first-line therapy is unlikely to be of benefit).

Q8

- Temporal (giant cell) arteritis (GCA) is an inflammatory condition that is associated with polymyalgia rheumatica, and this patient has clear symptoms of both. Visual symptoms would necessitate further investigation such as temporal artery biopsy.
- The patient would be expected to be on a reducing dose of prednisolone and may remain on them for 2 years or more.
- The patient should be issued with a steroid card and told to carry this on his person at all times in case of a medical emergency.
- The criteria for diagnosing GCA which include age, clinical signs, inflammatory markers and biopsy (8) were shown in 2012 to not be adequately predictive unless a biopsy was included.

The correct answer is:

Mark(s)	Criteria			Answer		
4	Optimal drug choice			*Prednisolone*		
4	Dosage	Route	Frequency	*60 mg*	*Oral*	*OD*
1	Timing			*Morning*		
1	Signature			*Signature*		

Sub-optimal choices for which the drug choice mark will be reduced are:

- Any drug other than prednisolone is unacceptable.
- The mark for this dose would be sub-optimal if less than 60 mg, and zero if more than 80 mg. This is because 60 mg is the preferred dose for an elderly patient due to the long-term side effects of steroids.

PRESCRIPTION REVIEW

Q1

The correct answer to Question A is lisinopril and methotrexate.

- Lisinopril is an ACE inhibitor (ACEI) and works by acting on the renin–angiotensin–aldosterone pathway. Its action results in an increase in bradykinin which is known to irritate the throat and cause a tickly cough.
- Methotrexate-induced pneumonitis can present as a dry cough, shortness of breath and, in advanced disease, with signs of cyanosis.

The correct answer to Question B is carvedilol and verapamil.

- The combination of a beta-blocker and verapamil carries the possible interaction of sudden hypotension and asystole. This could be in the acute setting with intravenous beta-blocker therapy or in the non-acute setting with oral treatment regimes.

Q2

The correct answer for Question A is digoxin.

- This question tests knowledge of medications causing interactions with warfarin and digoxin. Warfarin interactions occur largely through drug inhibition or induction of cytochrome P450 and effects on vitamin K metabolism and absorption.

The correct answers for Question B are amlodipine, bendroflumethiazide and spironolactone.

- Drugs cause digoxin toxicity via two routes; by prompting hypokalaemia or hypomagnesaemia (e.g. loop and thiazide diuretics), or by increasing plasma concentrations of digoxin (e.g. amiodarone, calcium channel blockers, spironolactone and quinine).

Q3

The correct answers for Question A are isosorbide mononitrate, tamsulosin and ramipril.

- Alpha-blockade (via tamsulosin), ACE inhibition (via ramipril) and venodilation (via isosorbide mononitrate) can lead to postural hypotension. Tamsulosin is the most likely agent to cause this side effect. Isosorbide mononitrate is a venodilator, so it can also cause sudden pooling of blood in the distal limbs and hence cause postural hypotension.

The correct answer for Question B is ferrous fumarate.

- Iron and calcium salts interact to reduce the efficacy of levothyroxine. For this reason they should be prescribed at a different time of day.

Q4
The correct answer for Question A is lithium.

- The patient is presenting with signs consistent with lithium toxicity, including cerebellar dysfunction (nystagmus and dysmetria), hyperthermia and hypernatraemia. Lithium is renally cleared and so the risk of toxicity is increased in the context of renal impairment.

The correct answers for Question B are bendroflumethiazide, furosemide and lithium.

- Loop and thiazide diuretics can lead to reduced sodium clearance and thus hypernatraemia.
- Lithium can cause nephrogenic diabetes insipidus (by inhibiting the action of antidiuretic hormone on the kidney) and lead to an increase in water wastage and increased serum osmolality as a result.

Q5
The correct answer for Question A is citalopram.

- A MHRA Drug Safety Update (Dec 2011) (9) set new restrictions on the maximum daily dose of citalopram due to the risk of prolonged Q–T syndrome. A 40 mg limit was set for adults and a 20 mg limit for patients older than 65 years or those with hepatic impairment.

The correct answers for Question B are amiodarone, citalopram and venlafaxine.

- Amiodarone and venlafaxine also interact to increase that risk in this patient, and for that reason even if the dose were corrected it would be sensible to arrange annual ECGs and check the BP and pulse as part of this patient's annual mental health review.

Q6
The correct answer for Question A is glibenclamide and metformin.

- The two prescriptions that are likely to be safe in pregnancy and breastfeeding are:
  - Glibenclamide is the only sulfonylurea recommended if breastfeeding (see BNF).
  - Metformin is used in gestational diabetes and is safe in pregnancy and breastfeeding.

- Of the other agents in the options list:
  - Aspirin should be avoided due to the possible risk of Reye's syndrome and also the association of its long-term use with impaired platelet function and risk of hypoprothrombinaemia in babies with low stores of vitamin K.

- Ciprofloxacin is a quinolone antibiotic which has been shown to cause arthropathy in animal models, thus it is not safe to use in pregnancy.
- Lisinopril is to be avoided as there is little information on its use in such conditions.

The correct answers for Question B are glibenclamide and metformin.

- The two agents that should be taken with food in order to be effective are the anti-diabetic agents glibenclamide and metformin.

Q7

The correct answer for Question A is clozapine.

- Clozapine belongs to a group of atypicial or second-generation antipsychotics. This group have a favourable adverse effect profile, particularly with regard to dopaminergic adverse effects, when compared to typical or first-generation antipsychotics. However, they are associated with disturbance in glucose metabolism and the development of the metabolic syndrome. The patient in this case is displaying symptoms of hyperosmolarity secondary to hyperglycaemia. The blurred vision is due to changes in the osmolarity of the vitreous and can be one of the first symptoms of diabetes.

The correct answers for Question B are paracetamol, doxycycline and digoxin.

- Paracetamol is prescribed in overdose with regard to the patient's BMI and should be 500 mg four times a day.
- Digoxin and doxycycline have been prescribed at loading doses.

Q8

The correct answer for Question A is atazanavir/ritonavir.

- Atazanavir and ritonavir are protease inhibitors and both are inhibitors of cytochrome P450. Ritonavir boosts the potency of atazanavir and so the drugs are delivered in combination.

The correct answers for Question B are allopurinol, carbamazepine and co-trimoxazole.

- DRESS (drug reaction with eosinophilia and systemic symptoms) syndrome is typically characterized by eosinophilia and systemic symptoms including fever, lymphadenopathy and liver dysfunction. It is an example of a delayed type IV hypersensitivity reaction and common precipitants include allopurinol, anti-epileptics and sulphonamides.

PLANNING MANAGEMENT

Q1
The correct answer is 'A'.

- This patient fulfils three out of four of Centor's criteria and as such should be prescribed antibiotics orally to treat a potential group A streptococcal infection.
- Intravenous treatment and ENT emergency admission are mainly indicated in cases of trismus or suspected quinsy.
- Advice regarding self-limiting viral illness should include self-management schemes through the local pharmacist.
- Throat swabs should not delay treatment in cases where bacterial infection is likely.
- Arranging a mono-spot test for glandular fever is an important consideration when ampicillin or amoxicillin is being considered, due to the risk of rash.

Q2
The correct answer is 'A'.

- The patient in this vignette has an ST-elevation myocardial infarction (STEMI) and thus requires primary coronary intervention (PCI). However, prior to this, they should receive a loading dose of aspirin. A further anti-platelet may be added, but the use of aspirin is so important that it is usually given pre-hospital.
- The other medications should be commenced (unless contraindicated) but are not the first to be given.

Q3
The correct answer is 'D'.

- This patient has presented with symptoms of hyperglycaemia which causes polydipsia and polyuria as a result of osmotic effects on the circulation, and blurring of vision due to osmotic effects within the eye.
- The patient is also overweight and so would benefit from treatment with metformin as first line. However, his renal function should be checked prior to commencing metformin as it is renally cleared and may increase the risk of lactic acidosis in the context of renal impairment.

Q4
The correct answer is 'E'.

- It is always important to establish why a patient is taking anti-coagulation. If it is for atrial fibrillation, the anti-coagulation is to act as stroke prophylaxis. If it is for a pulmonary embolus or metallic valvular prosthesis, it is to stop them from clotting off one of the patient's great vessels.

Obviously, the risks of missed anti-coagulation are more significant in the latter two examples.

- If a patient begins to bleed, especially leading to haemodynamic instability, the reversal of anti-coagulation must be pursued. In this case, it is important to reverse the patient's anti-coagulation with vitamin K (intravenously), and prothrombin complex may also be considered. The platelets are not low enough to necessitate replacement (usually if <60 and bleeding). A cross-match should also be taken and O negative blood can be used if a cross-match would take too long.

Q5

The correct answer is 'C'.

- The diagnosis is acute PID. The NICE guidelines (2015) (10) state that patients with PID can be treated in primary care with a combination of oral and intramuscular antibiotics; however, when the patient has certain clinical markers, they should be admitted.
- In this case, the patient has severe pain and vomiting, a significant pyrexia and tenderness on PV, as well as raised inflammatory markers. Empirical antibiotics are recommended to cover chlamydia, *Neisseria* and also anaerobes.
- Appendicitis and ectopic pregnancy are viable differential diagnoses but can be excluded by the history and examination in some cases.

Q6

The correct answer is 'B'.

- This is a typical history for a corneal abrasion. Eye patches are no longer recommended as they are not shown to reduce the rate of healing or reduce the symptoms of pain. Artificial tears may be required after the initial week of prophylactic antibiotics.
- Local anaesthetic drops such as amethocaine should not be given to patients for self-administering.
- Missing a penetrating eye injury is one of the commonest causes of litigation with eye trauma cases; however, the history is usually one of a flying small object, for example due to power tool use.
- Contact lenses should not be worn until 24 hours after the last day of antibiotics.

Q7

The correct answer is 'C'.

- At this stage, it is better to manage the patient's presenting complaint and liaise with the surgical team for an elective admission only if a laparotomy or another procedure is required.

- The patient is dehydrated as can be seen from the clinical presentation and subsequent blood results. It is thus important to rehydrate and rectify any electrolyte imbalance as the first priority.
- IV antibiotics will be needed especially if, as the WCC suggests, this patient has an infection. An anti-emetic agent will also be useful given this patient's presenting complaint. However, use of morphine may lead to a worsening of the pain. A better choice would be to use an anti-inflammatory agent.

Q8
The correct answer is 'D'.

- The presence of blood in the brain in acute subarachnoid haemorrhage causes inflammation and therefore vasoconstriction of cerebral blood vessels.
- The medical management of choice is to commence the calcium channel blocker nimodipine which is known to penetrate the brain better than other drugs in this class.

COMMUNICATING INFORMATION

Q1

The correct answer is 'C'.

Option A	Codeine is an opioid analgesic; its most likely side effects are nausea, vomiting, drowsiness and constipation.
Option B	Metronidazole is an antibacterial agent most effective against anaerobic microorganisms.
Option C	Codeine (as well as metronidazole) can cause drowsiness.
Option D	It is better to take paracetamol regularly in order to help resolve the pain. Taking this medication PRN will make it less effective in this instance.
Option E	It is not safe to consume alcohol while on this set of medication because of the additive drowsiness effect and interaction with metronidazole.

Q2

The correct answer is 'C'.

Option A	Avoidance of exercise late in the day is preferred to help improve sleep patterns.
Option B	A reduction in intake of alcohol, spicy food, caffeine and tobacco may be helpful in improving hot flushes.
Option C	Regular exercise will help with hot flushes as well as sleep pattern. Losing weight may also reduce the frequency and severity of flushes, as there is evidence that a BMI >30 kg/m^2 can increase the likelihood of flushing.
Option D	Transdermal HRT may be of use in this patient if lifestyle modifications do not help.
Option E	Having a regular bedtime is more likely to help improve sleep patterns.

Q3

The correct answer is 'D'.

Option A	If two consecutive pills are missed in the first week of the pack and the patient has had sexual intercourse since the beginning of the pill-free week, then emergency contraception should be given.
Option B	The guidance in the pill packet inserts may well still state the previous rules – that a missed pill meant it had not been taken within 12 hours of the usual time.
Option C	The guidance now (MHRA, 2011) (11) is that a missed pill is defined as one forgotten by more than 24 hours. If this is the case, then two should be taken when remembered.
Option D	If two consecutive pills are missed anywhere in the pack, then the guidance states to take extra precautions for 7 days.
Option E	If two consecutive pills are missed in week 3, then the guidance states to omit the pill-free week.

- This patient has missed two of her combined contraceptive pills on consecutive days. The guidance for missed pills has changed in the past few years.
- The guidance now (MHRA, 2011) (11) is that a missed pill is defined as one forgotten by more than 24 hours. If this is the case, then two should be taken when remembered.
- If two consecutive pills are missed anywhere in the pack, then the guidance states:
  - Take the second missed pill with the pill that was due.
  - Take extra precautions for 7 days.
  - Omit the pill-free week if the two pills were forgotten in the preceding week.

Q4
The correct answer is 'A'.

Option A	In an infant, use of steroid around the eyes should be avoided in general, although mild-potency hydrocortisone can be used in some cases.
Option B	Emollients are of limited benefit in an acute flare-up, although have a role to play in longer term maintenance, but there is a risk of folliculitis if applied in more directions than just in the direction of hair growth.
Option C	Overexposure to water removes the natural protective function of skin, even with emollient bath additives which are not shown to be of much benefit.
Option D	Pimecrolimus can be used in a child <2 years old, but this is initiated by a specialist only.
Option E	Stepping up to a moderate-potency steroid is sometimes necessary for 1–2 weeks.

Q5
The correct answer is 'A'.

Option A	Isotretinoin is teratogenic and contraception is mandatory in sexually active females.
Option B	Hyperlipidaemia and hepatitis are potential side effects of isotretinoin.
Option C	A possible link exists between isotretinoin and suicidal ideations.
Option D	There is a potential risk of pancreatitis with hypertriglyceridaemia.
Option E	Isotretinoin works by inhibiting sebum production.

- Counselling is very important when commencing on isotretinoin, and in practice most of the above should be touched on or monitored for; however, the most important piece of information for a sexually active teenager to convey is the pregnancy prevention issue.

Q6
The correct answer is 'D'.

Option A	Doses of iron and calcium supplements should be taken 4 hours apart from levothyroxine.
Option B	Thyroid function is usually reviewed 3 months after a change in therapy.
Option C	Liver problems due to carbimazole are rare.
Option D	This could be indicative of agranulocytosis which has been associated with fatalities.
Option E	Folic acid supplementation is not particularly required for carbimazole therapy.

CALCULATIONS

Q1

Correct answer

170 mg (171 mg accepted)

Working

First establish whether the renal function is adequate for the patient to receive gentamicin using the Cockcroft–Gault equation:

Estimated creatinine clearance in men
$$= \{[140 - \text{Age (years)} \times \text{Mass (kg)}] \times 1.23/[(\text{Serum Cr (micromol/L)}]\}$$
In women, the answer is multiplied by 0.85.

Thus: $[(140 - 85) \times 57 \times 1.23]/120$
$$= 3856/120$$
$$= 32 \text{ mL/min}$$
As we have a female patient, we need to add in the final factor:
$32 \times 0.85 = 27.3$ mL/min

This is greater than 20 mL/min, so the patient can receive gentamicin based on her renal function.

To calculate the dose of gentamicin:

3 mg/kg × 57 kg = 171 mg (this should be rounded to 170 mg)

Q2

Correct answer

2 L (2016 is actual answer)

Working

$1.2 \times 70 = 84$
$84 \times 24 = 2016$ (i.e. 2 × 1-L bags)

- The aim of fluid replacement post-surgery in part is to avoid crystalloid excess (e.g. sodium chloride and water overload). Maintenance fluid when utilized is usually given at 2 mL/kg/h or less, and this is inclusive of any drug infusions.
- The use of an isotonic electrolyte solution is preferred (such as Hartmann's solution) as it will minimize the risk of hyperchloraemic acidosis.
- For more information on this topic, a useful reference source can be reviewed (12).

Q3

Correct answer

325 mg or 650 mg

Working

Dose = 250 mg/m^2 or 500 mg/m^2

BSA = 1.3 (as per table at the back of the BNF for children, or BNFC)

Dose = 250 × BSA
  = 250 × 1.3
  = 325 mg

OR

Dose = 500 × BSA
  = 500 × 1.3
  = 650 mg

Q4

Correct answer

8 drops

Working

See BNF section 4.3.3 under 'citalopram monograph'.

4 drops (8 mg) ≡ 10 mg tablet dose

Many prescribers will unwittingly prescribe 10 drops.

Q5

Correct answer

224 or 240 tablets

Working

See BNF section 5.1.9, under 'Rifampicin, combined preparations'.
The initial phase is 2 months in duration.
Dose for a patient weighing 55–70 kg is 4 tablets daily.
4 × 28 × 2 = 224
OR
4 × 30 × 2 = 240
As the product comes in a pack size of 60 tablets, it is best to keep to multiples of this number.
For this reason 240 is a better choice.

Q6

Correct answer

156 mg

Working

Dose = 78 × 2 = 156 mg
(Note use of booking weight)
For more information on HIV infection in pregnant woman, refer to BHIVA guidance, available
  online (13).

Q7

Correct answer

59 tablets

Working

40 mg OM for 7/7 → 8 × 7 = 56
30 mg OM for 5/7 → 6 × 5 = 30
20 mg OM for 5/7 → 4 × 5 = 20
10 mg OM for 3/7 → 2 × 3 = 6
5 mg OM for 3/7 → 1 × 3 = 3

Patient already has 56 tablets.
Hence you only need to request a further 59 tablets in order for her to complete the course.

Q8

Correct answer

60 mg (the dose needs to be rounded from 62.5 mg)

Working

You are told that prednisolone 5 mg ≡ methylprednisolone 4 mg.

You are also told that the patient commences on 50 mg of methylprednisolone.

50/4 = 12.5

12.5 × 5 = 62.5 mg

In reality this would be rounded to 60 mg.

ADVERSE DRUG REACTIONS

Q1 (Type A)
The correct answer is 'B'.

- Tolterodine is an anticholinergic drug that works by blocking the muscarinic receptors and therefore has anticholinergic side effects.
- Of these side effects, a dry mouth is the most commonly experienced in practice. GI side effects are the next likely and this includes constipation. Urinary retention is rare, but some problems with urine are possible. CNS side effects are more likely in the elderly, such as agitation and confusion.
- Bladder retraining should also be a key management option in a patient of this age.

Q2 (Type B)
The correct answer is 'D'.

- Mirtazapine is a newer generation antidepressant that works by increasing the neurotransmission of serotonin and noradrenaline centrally, therefore having the same outcome as an SNRI but by a more direct mechanism.
- It is well known for causing weight gain, which is a common disadvantage and reason for intolerance in many patients.
- It is best taken at night as it induces drowsiness, which helps a lot of patients with depression with symptoms of poor sleep (although this only lasts in the early stages after initiation).

Q3 (Type C)
The correct answer is 'D'.

- Citalopram when prescribed alongside a non-steroidal anti-inflammatory drug (NSAID) will lead to an increased risk of gastro-intestinal bleeding. It is possible to use it short term or minimize the risk of this by adding a gastro-protective agent.

Q4 (Type D)
The correct answer is 'A'.

- The symptoms are suggestive of a number of differential diagnoses, for example diverticulitis, IBS, acute appendicitis and ulceration, among others. It is also plausible that the medication he is using has nothing to do with the sickness and pain and that they are due to his underlying condition.
- Use of an NSAID may not be warranted long term as it can lead to diverticular perforation and/or increase the risk of GI ulceration and bleeding. This patient also has a background which suggests an NSAID may not be the most appropriate drug choice. For these reasons, it is best to stop diclofenac.

Q5 (Type A)
The correct answer is 'E'.

- Hydroxychloroquine is a good treatment for inflammatory arthropathy, with a very acceptable adverse effect profile. However, hydroxychloroquine-associated retinopathy is a rare but important adverse effect that should be considered in patients presenting with a change in vision.
- The Royal College of Optometrists has provided guidance on how to prevent ocular toxicity in those on long-term treatment (14). This includes the recording of near-vision acuity prior to and periodically during treatment using a Snellen chart and referral to an ophthalmologist if any changes in visual acuity occur.
- It is also important to note that ocular toxicity is less likely where the drug dosage is based on ideal body weight in obese patients.
- Where the dose is less than 4 mg/kg/day of chloroquine phosphate (equivalent to 2.5 mg/kg/day of chloroquine base), ocular toxicity is unlikely to occur.

Q6 (Type B)
The correct answer is 'E'.

- Calcium channel blockers are known to cause flushing and headaches. This effect can be negated by lowering the dose and/or switching to an alternative if this does not help.

Q7 (Type C)
The correct answer is 'B'.

- This is a common interaction that has in some cases led to fatalities. It is advised to withhold the statin while on clarithromycin therapy.
- Concomitant use with certain drugs will also necessitate caution in terms of dosing. For this reason, choosing amlodipine is not the correct option as this interaction has been mitigated to an extent with use of lower doses of both interacting agents.
- For more information on this topic, review Ref. (15).
- In some cases, simvastatin can be switched to atorvastatin (which has a lower propensity for this interaction) for secondary prevention or pravastatin (which does not carry this interaction) for primary prevention.
- It is advised that the calcium channel blocker is not changed as this is clinically less desirable, especially in cases where the patient's condition is well controlled on their current therapy.

Q8 (Type D)
The correct answer is 'C'.

- The combination of a pustular rash and neutrophilia as manifestations of a drug reaction point towards a diagnosis of acute generalized exanthematous pustulosis (AGEP).
- AGEP is a severe cutaneous adverse drug reaction often – though not exclusively – occurring secondary to antibiotic therapy. The common candidates include penicillin-based antibiotics and sulphonamides, such as trimethoprim.
- AGEP can be associated with liver function derangement.
- Another important severe cutaneous drug reaction to recognize is DRESS syndrome, which includes fever and liver function derangement. Treatment is a combination of stopping the offending drug and managing symptoms.

DRUG MONITORING

Q1
The correct answer is 'C'.

- Changes in blood pressure may be expected due to the mode of action of caffeine; this will not allow us to gauge if the child is having too much drug.
- Although monitoring heart rate is useful, it will not give us any further information as to the amount of drug that is leading to this increase.
- TDM levels are necessary as this child is exhibiting signs of caffeine toxicity. A trough level is needed and levels should be in the range of 5–25 mg/L; in cases where levels are >30 mg/L, toxicity may be expected.
- Urinary output is a good indicator with nephrotoxic drugs or drugs that are highly water soluble. This is not the case with caffeine.
- Looking at this child's weight will allow you to determine if the dose is appropriate but will not give you any further information needed to determine your next course of action.

Q2
The correct answer is 'A'.

- The best way to monitor for the effects of fluid replacement is to keep a check on the patient's blood pressure and urine output, as this will allow you to gauge the response to fluid intake as well as allow you to ensure the patient is not overloaded with fluid.
- A full blood count and urea and electrolyte values are not a necessity in this instance, unless we needed to look at such parameters in cases where infection is suspected or there has been significant blood loss.
- Oxygen saturations are not useful in this instance unless it is suspected the patient is fluid overloaded, in which case it is useful to check the respiratory rate too.

Q3
The correct answer is 'D'.

- Hepatic encephalopathy occurs due to an inability of the diseased liver to excrete ammonia, which therefore builds up in the blood and manifests neurotoxic effects. In the case of the patient described above, this presented as confusion or delirium.
- Constipation leads to an increased absorption of ammonia from the lumen of the bowel and so can precipitate an encephalopathic presentation. The treatment is lactulose, with the addition of phosphate enemas if required if bowel motions are not stimulated. It is therefore vital to monitor the stool chart.

Q4

The correct answer is 'C'.

- The patient in this case has bacterial meningitis. The most important clinical monitoring parameter is the Glasgow coma score (GCS), as this provides information on sepsis and cerebral function as a result of meningeal inflammation and swelling.

Q5

The correct answer is 'C'.

- The most likely adverse effect is bradycardia, which will be seen with a pulse lower than 60 bpm. It is important to note that digoxin must be withheld if the pulse falls below 60 bpm.
- Disturbances in potassium and magnesium levels characterized by a drop in either of these two parameters can lead to digitalis toxicity.
- Visual field test are not necessary, but it is important to note that digoxin can cause neurological disturbances including blurred vision and yellow vision (characterized by yellow–green halos).

Q6

The correct answer is 'D'.

- Venlafaxine is a serotonin and noradrenaline reuptake inhibitor. At higher doses, especially at 300 mg and above, it is known to carry a risk of elevating blood pressure and also prolonged Q-T syndrome. This risk is higher in those with pre-existing heart disease or hypertension; therefore, it is essential to monitor these parameters on a regular basis, at least annually.

Q7

The correct answer is 'B'.

- Azathioprine is a thiopurine immunosuppressant which acts through T cell modulation.
- It is associated with hepatotoxicity and bone marrow suppression, and as such requires monitoring of full blood count and liver function testing.
- It is also important to check thiopurine methyltransferase (TPMT) levels prior to commencement as this affects the metabolism of the drug and the risk of toxicity.

Q8
The correct answer is 'E'.

- Lithium has a narrow therapeutic index of 0.5–1.2 mmol/L taken 12 hours after a dose. NICE guidelines (16) state that this should be done every 3 months. Lithium also has renal and thyroid toxicity effects, and NICE recommends that renal and thyroid function should be checked every 6 months for these patients.
- This is more stringent than the current QOF targets in general practice, which allow lithium levels to be checked every 4 months and thyroid and renal function to be checked annually.

DATA INTERPRETATION

Q1
The correct answer is 'E'.

- This patient has considerable cardiovascular risk.
- This is calculated by using a validated CVD risk calculator and can be accessed through the eBNF (http://qrisk.org).
- These risk scores are designed for use in primary prevention cases as opposed to secondary prevention.
- Diabetics should not be considered for risk assessment scores as they are considered equivalent to having had a cardiovascular event, provided they are >50 years old or have had diabetes for >10 years (17).

Q2
The correct answer is 'C'.

- This patient is showing signs of sepsis; there is expert consensus that if such a patient is admitted to hospital, he/she is treated with an intravenous carbapenem-based antibiotic (especially in those recently hospitalized or with recurrent UTIs). Where an oral antibiotic is indicated, the drug of choice would be ciprofloxacin, cefalexin or co-amoxiclav depending on the clinical profile of the patient (e.g. allergy status).
- A midstream urine sample is needed for culture and sensitivity before starting empirical antibiotics. Any pain and/or fever will need treatment and full hydration must be maintained.
- The patient should be reviewed within 24 hours to assess response to treatment and to review the clinical picture. Use of intravenous antibiotics should help to improve the patient in this time frame.
- Referral to investigate any underlying renal tract anatomical or functional abnormality (such as vesico-ureteric reflux and polycystic kidney disease) is generally needed in:
  - Men who present for the first time with acute pyelonephritis
  - Women following two or more episodes of acute pyelonephritis
  - All patients with Proteus-based UTIs
- For more information on this topic, review Ref. (18).

Q3
The correct answer is 'E'.

- Ramipril is an ACE-1 inhibitor and is known to cause renal toxicity. This is more likely when there is silent reno-vascular disease, and it is very risky in the presence of bilateral renal artery stenosis.
- In such cases the possibility of reduced or even abolished glomerular filtration is greater.
- This patient has a history of PVD, so the chances of atherosclerotic disease affecting the renal arteries are higher.

Q4

The correct answer is 'C'.

- Beta-blockers can cause IUGR, neonatal hypoglycaemia and bradycardia; this risk is greater in severe hypertension. Labetalol is said to be the safest option.
- ACEIs are largely avoided in pregnancy as they can affect foetal BP control and renal capacity. In some case reports, oligohydramnios and skull defects have also been reported.
- Labetalol is the safest choice in pregnancy due to it having the greater clinical evidence base.
- Methyldopa is considered to be safe in pregnancy but must be stopped within 2 days of birth and the patient switched back to their original anti-hypertensive.
- Nifedipine is an option but may inhibit labour. It is generally not used before week 20 of the pregnancy. The risk to the foetus versus the benefit to mum should be evaluated before using this drug. It is only used where other treatment options have failed or are no longer indicated.

Q5

The correct answer is 'C'.

- The key to answering questions on calcium metabolism is in understanding the key players: vitamin D and PTH.
- PTH causes calcium to rise and phosphate to drop.
- Vitamin D causes calcium and phosphate to rise.
- In the case in question, vitamin D is being given and so should be held initially while further investigations are ongoing.

Q6

The correct answer is 'E'.

- Pregnancy is a pro-diabetogenic state. All pregnant women are therefore screened for gestational diabetes.
- The risk factors for gestational diabetes include family history of diabetes; South Asian, black Caribbean or Middle Eastern ethnic origin; previous gestational diabetes; obesity; BMI >30; and a previous macrosomic baby.
- The screening test is an oral glucose tolerance test (GTT) at 28 weeks.
- Treatment can include oral metformin or long-acting/fast-acting insulin as well as blood glucose monitoring and lifestyle advice. Other hypoglycaemic agent medications are contraindicated in pregnancy.

PSA Paper Two – Answers and Rationale

PRESCRIBING

Q1

The correct answer is:

Mark(s)	Criteria			Answer		
4	Optimal drug choice			Glucose 50% and insulin (Actrapid®)		
4	Dosage	Route	Frequency	50 mL with 10–12 units	Intravenous	Once only
1	Timing			STAT		
1	Signature			Signature		

- Hyperkalaemia is a common medical emergency, and it is therefore incredibly important to have a working grasp of its management.
- This patient has already received calcium gluconate to stabilize the myocardium; however, they still require insulin dextrose in the form of Actrapid 10–12 units + 50 mL of 50% glucose.
- This will drive potassium out of the systemic circulation and into cells.
- Salbutamol may be used (unless contraindicated); however, it is simply a secondary measure.

Sub-optimal choices for which the drug choice mark will be reduced are:

- Salbutamol – 2 marks awarded out of 4 (as this will promote hypokalaemia but is not always first line).
- Intravenous fluid not containing potassium (e.g. 0.9% sodium chloride, glucose) – 1 mark awarded out of 4.

Q2

The correct answer is:

Mark(s)	Criteria			Answer		
4	Optimal drug choice			Heparin (unfractionated)		
4	Dosage	Route	Frequency	5000 units	Subcutaneous	Twice daily
1	Timing			0800 and 1800		
1	Signature			Signature		

- All patients admitted to hospital are at an increased risk of venous thromboemboli. In this patient's case the risk will be increased as her urinary sepsis will lead to the release of prothrombotic inflammatory mediators including fibrinogen and a likely reduction in her mobility state.
- Because of this risk, thromboprophylaxis should always be considered and prescribed when required (as in the case above).
- Low-molecular-weight heparin is the usual choice for patient with a normal renal function, and bear in mind that obese patients may require higher doses.
- This patient has impaired renal function and so the low-molecular-weight heparin (which is cleared in the urine) would build up, leading to higher levels than intended.
- For this reason, **unfractionated subcutaneous heparin should be prescribed at 5000 units twice daily**. The two doses are usually given 12 hours apart with the evening dose at 1800 so that a 'round of thromboprophylaxis' can be administered by nursing staff.

Sub-optimal choices for which the drug choice mark will be reduced are:

- The prescribing of a low-molecular-weight heparin (e.g. dalteparin), in the context of impaired renal function, would result in unpredictable pharmacodynamics and so should receive 0 marks out of the 4 awarded.

Q3
The correct answer is:

Mark(s)	Criteria			Answer		
4	Optimal drug choice			Naloxone		
4	Dosage	Route	Frequency	0.4–2 mg	Intravenous	Once only
1	Timing			STAT		
1	Signature			Signature		

- The presence of 1 mm pupils bilaterally (or 'pin-point pupils'), a reduced level of consciousness and a reduced respiratory rate (respiratory depression) within the context of substance misuse should guide you to a diagnosis of opiate overdose, the treatment for which is naloxone.
- Naloxone is an opiate receptor antagonist and can work incredibly quickly, leading to the patient suddenly becoming very alert and, often, very aggressive.
- Naloxone should be prescribed initially as an intravenous injection of 0.4–2 mg and repeated every 2–3 minutes until there is a response (to a maximum of 10 mg).
- An infusion of 60% of the total dose required to produce a response per hour is then given. It is important to monitor for a prolonged period in long-acting preparations such as methadone.

Sub-optimal choices for which the drug choice mark will be reduced are:

- Oxygen – 3 marks awarded out of 4.

Q4

The correct answer is:

Mark(s)	Criteria			Answer		
4	Optimal drug choice			*Levonorgestrel*		
4	Dosage	Route	Frequency	*1.5 mg*	*Oral*	*Once only*
1	Timing			*STAT*		
1	Signature			*Signature*		

- The MAP (morning-after pill) is one option for emergency contraception.
- The above preparation is only effective if given within 72 hours of UPSI.
- The failure rate is approximately 1 in 8, but the failure is more likely to occur in the 48–72 hour window.
- Nausea can occur after either levenorgestrel or ulipristal and it will need to be taken again if this occurs within 2 and 3 hours of administration, respectively.

Sub-optimal choices for which the drug choice mark will be reduced are:

- Levonelle-2® – 3 marks awarded out of 4 (non-generic prescribing should not be routine).
- Copper IUCD – 2 marks awarded out of 4 (this may be an option in a 21 year old, depending on her personal choice and plans for her future family).
- Ullipristal – 1 mark awarded out of 4 (this should not be first line unless the time post UPSI is 3–5 days).

Q5

The correct answer is:

Mark(s)	Criteria			Answer		
4	Optimal drug choice			*Amoxicillin*		
4	Dosage	Route	Frequency	*500 mg*	*Oral*	*TDS*
1	Timing			*8 hours apart*		
1	Signature			*Signature*		

Sub-optimal choices for which the drug choice mark will be reduced are:

- Clarithromycin 250 or 500 mg BD – 3 marks awarded out of 4 (as no penicillin allergy stated).
- Doxycycline 200 mg STAT, then 100 mg daily – 3 marks awarded out of 4 (as no penicillin allergy stated).
- Co-amoxiclav 625 mg TDS – 2 marks awarded out of 4 (usually a second-line antibiotic due to higher risk of side effects, mainly cholestatic jaundice).

Q6

The correct answer options are:

Mark(s)	Criteria			Answer		
4	Optimal drug choice			Clarithromycin		
4	Dosage	Route	Frequency	125 mg	Oral	BD
1	Timing			12 hours apart		
1	Signature			Signature		

Mark(s)	Criteria			Answer		
4	Optimal drug choice			Erythromycin		
4	Dosage	Route	Frequency	250 mg OR 500 mg	Oral	QDS OR BD
1	Timing			6 hours apart OR 12 hours apart		
1	Signature			Signature		

- This child has presented with impetigo (as confirmed by the swab results).
- The mainstay of treatment is usually flucloxacillin ± phenoxymethyl-penicillin in severe cases. However, this child has an allergy to penicillin, the nature of which would need to be determined.
- Alternative agents in penicillin allergic patients are macrolide antibiotics such as:
  - Clarithromycin at a dose of 125 mg BD for 7 days
  - Azithromycin at a dose of 200 mg OD for 3 days
  - Erythromycin at a dose of 250 mg QDS or 500 mg BD (as a total daily dose can be given in two divided doses)
- Topical fusidic acid can be prescribed if small areas of skin are affected, or mupirocin (if MRSA suspected); however, topical treatments are not recommended as much due to increasing resistance, and where prescribed they should not be used for longer than 10 days.
- Clindamycin is another suitable agent if susceptible organisms are isolated, but it is not first line.
- For more details and a sample scenario on managing impetigo, please see Ref. (19).

Sub-optimal choices for which the drug choice mark will be reduced are:

- Azithromycin – 3 marks awarded out of 4 (suitable alternative but not first choice as it is more useful in atypical respiratory infections).
- Topical treatment – 2 marks awarded out of 4 (not recommended due to increasing resistance).
- Clindamycin – 1 mark awarded out of 4 (not first line).

Q7
The correct answer is:

Mark(s)	Criteria			Answer		
4	Optimal drug choice			*Isphagula husk*		
4	Dosage	Route	Frequency	*1 sachet*	*Oral*	*BD*
1	Timing			*After meals (not immediately before going to bed)*		
1	Signature			*Signature*		

- This patient is 33 weeks pregnant, so this will affect our choice of laxative.
- The first choice in such a patient is a bulk-forming laxative such as isphagula husk. However, bear in mind this is not suitable if the patient has had chronic constipation (lasting over 6 months), is suspected to have faecal impaction or has inadequate fluid intake.
- The full effect of bulk-forming laxatives may take a few days to develop. Patients should be told that they need to take them with water and not immediately before retiring to bed.
- Second-line agents are usually an osmotic laxative with or without a stimulant laxative. A good example is prescribing macrogol with senna.
- Where treatment has failed with the above two options, consider specialist referral as other medication may be needed (e.g. prucalopride).
- For more information on constipation in pregnancy, please refer to the NICE guidance on constipation (20).

Sub-optimal choices for which the drug choice mark will be reduced are:

- Methylcellulose or sterculia granules = 3 marks awarded out of 4 (as these preparations are not as cost effective).
- Osmotic laxative ± stimulant laxative = 2 marks awarded out of 4.
- Rectal enema = 1 mark awarded out of 4 (due to risk of electrolyte disturbances and by virtue of them not being first line).

Q8
The correct answer options are:

Mark(s)	Criteria			Answer		
4	Optimal drug choice			*Glyceryl tri-nitrate 400 microgram spray*		
4	Dosage	Route	Frequency	*1 or 2 puffs*	*S/L*	*STAT*
1	Timing			*Immediately*		
1	Signature			*Signature*		

Mark(s)	Criteria			Answer		
4	Optimal drug choice			*Glyceryl tri-nitrate 500 microgram S/L tabs*		
4	Dosage	Route	Frequency	*1 tablet*	*S/L*	*STAT*
1	Timing			*Immediately*		
1	Signature			*Signature*		

Rationale:

- This man has presented with signs of unstable angina which will respond to a quick-acting nitro-vasodilator such as glyceryl tri-nitrate. For more information, see Ref. (21).

Sub-optimal choices for which the drug choice mark will be reduced are:

- Morphine – 2 marks awarded out of 4.
- Oxygen – 1 mark awarded out of 4.

PRESCRIPTION REVIEW

Q1

The correct answer to Question A is omeprazole.

- Gastric protection should always be considered in patients receiving dual anti-platelet therapy; however, the preference is for lansoprazole or ranitidine, as omeprazole interacts unfavourably with clopidogrel to reduce efficacy.
- Clopidogrel is a pro-drug and is converted to active metabolites. This conversion is impaired by omeprazole and esomeprazole.

The correct answers to Question B are furosemide, metformin and ramipril.

- The acute kidney injury in this case could be secondary to reduced perfusion within the context of a myocardial infarction, contrast nephropathy or drug-induced acute kidney injury. The question asks for three medications that are most likely to contribute to the acute kidney injury. These are:
  - Furosemide, a loop diuretic used in the treatment of cardiac failure. It can improve dyspnoea in patients with pulmonary oedema by offloading fluid from the systemic circulation. However, in the context of acute kidney injury, the use of diuretics should be carefully considered with a harm–benefit analysis.
  - Ramipril, an ACE inhibitor (ACEI) that inhibits efferent arteriole vasoconstriction in the glomerulus. This leads to a reduction in the pressure difference across the glomerulus and thus a reduction in blood flow. Eventually this can lead to acute kidney injury and acute tubular necrosis.
  - Metformin, a bi-guanide that is renally cleared and in the context of acute kidney injury may accumulate, leading to an increased risk of lactic acidosis.

Q2

The correct answer to Question A is omeprazole, amoxicillin and sodium valproate.

- The above medications are inhibitors of cytochrome P450, leading to a reduction in the metabolism of warfarin and thus an increase in warfarin levels in the systemic circulation. In the above patient this has led to an increase in the INR.

The correct answer to Question B is lamotrigine.

- Lamotrigine (more than sodium valproate) is associated with cutaneous adverse effects, including those on the spectrum from erythema multiforme to Stevens–Johnson syndrome to toxic epidermal necrolysis. The treatment of generalized epilepsy is initially sodium valproate with another anticonvulsant (in this case lamotrigine) added in for resistant disease.

Q3

The correct answer to Question A is carbamazepine, rifabutin and griseofulvin.

- All anticonvulsants of the older generation except sodium valproate are liver enzyme inducers and so interact with the OCP. Newer anticonvulsants such as lamotrigine are not liver inducers but still interact and so should be avoided.
- Rifabutin is an antituberculosis drug and contains rifampicin, which STRONGLY interacts with the COCP (combined oral contraceptive pill) as it is a liver inducer too.
- Griseofulvin has also been reported to result in contraceptive failure and menstrual irregularities.

The correct answer to Question B is levothyroxine.

- The usual dose for levothyroxine is 100–125 micrograms.
- A dose of 200 micrograms is therefore far from this range.
- This is sometimes seen in practice due to a mistaken interpretation of a thyroid function test when the patient is actually just poorly compliant and has taken an erratic dosage prior to the test.

Q4

The correct answer to Question A is ramipril.

- Ramipril and other ACEIs are prone to cause postural hypotension; therefore, it is better to start off on a low dose (2.5 mg) and titrate up according to response to BP and the individual tolerability of the patient.

The correct answers to Question B are carbamazepine, bendroflumethiazide and fluoxetine.

- Carbamazepine is a common anti-epileptic but is relatively unknown for causing low sodium, whereas thiazide diuretics are a VERY common cause of a low sodium, as they inhibit sodium reabsorption at the DCT (although if it is <125, then consider non-iatrogenic causes such as Addison's disease and SIADH).
- SSRIs such as fluoxetine are also a potential cause of low sodium.

Other important issues around the drugs in this question are:

- Metformin (the only available bi-guanide) works by decreasing gluconeogenesis and by increasing peripheral utilization of glucose; therefore, it can be prescribed alongside insulin. It is the first-line hypoglycaemic agent when BMI >25.

- Carbamazepine can cause a yellow discoloration of skin that is possible to confuse for jaundice.

Q5

The correct answer to Question A is bisoprolol.

- This man has asthma. Bisoprolol is a beta-blocker and so it is contraindicated. Beta blockade can inhibit bronchial smooth muscle and therefore trigger the muscle contraction and could precipitate asthma attacks.
- Although bisoprolol is cardio-selective, it is not exclusively active on cardiac muscle only.

The correct answers to Question B are aspirin, bendroflumethiazide, and ramipril.

- This man's symptoms of a non-traumatic, exquisitely tender big toe are diagnostic of a gout attack.
- Gout is caused by uric acid crystals accumulating in joints, typically in the hallux first metatarsophalangeal.
- Aspirin is an NSAID and can precipitate gout attacks.
- Ramipril is an ACE-1 inhibitor and can also trigger gout.
- Thiazide diuretics can also precipitate gout.

Q6

The correct answer to Question A is lisinopril.

- Lisinopril is an ACEI and works by acting on the renin–angiotensin–aldosterone pathway. Its action results in an increase in bradykinin which is known to irritate the throat and cause a tickly cough.

The correct answer to Question B is carvedilol, gliclazide and verapamil.

- The combination of a beta-blocker and verapamil carries the possible interaction of sudden hypotension and asystole.
- This could be in the acute setting with IV beta-blocker, or in the non-acute setting with oral treatments.
- Gliclazide can also cause pre-syncope/dizziness by causing hypoglycaemia. Gliclazide, the most commonly prescribed sulfonylurea, works by forcing the pancreas to increase insulin secretion and therefore needs endogenous insulin capability. Sulfonylureas do have risks of hypoglycaemia, but gliclazide is less risky as it is shorter acting.

Q7

The correct answer to Question A is aspirin and ramipril.

- Aspirin and ACEIs are generally stopped one week before surgery due to risk of haemodynamic instability such as hypotension and increase in vasoconstriction requirements post-surgery. There may be some instances in high-risk patients where aspirin is not stopped.

The correct answer to Question B is gliclazide and metformin.

- Gliclazide must be omitted on the morning of surgery, and some guidance will specify to omit metformin too.
- In patients with hypertension, anaesthesia and surgery may increase heart rate and blood pressure. Beta-blockers will help suppress these effects and reduce cardiovascular complications (such as myocardial infarction) and are therefore usually continued peri-operatively.

Q8

The correct answer to Question A is aspirin.

- Aspirin is an obvious potential cause of the GI bleeding.
- The withholding of anti-platelet therapy may require discussion with a cardiologist, particularly in the context of coronary stenting, as if anti-platelets are discontinued too proximally to stent insertion, stent thrombosis may occur.

The correct answer to Question B is amitriptyline, bisoprolol and chlorphenamine.

- Amitriptyline, bisoprolol and chlorphenamine can all cause dry eyes and sicca symptoms.
- This occurs through inhibition of aqueous production, either directly or via an anti-muscarinic effect.

PLANNING MANAGEMENT

Q1
The correct answer is 'E'.

- This patient has a pulmonary embolus secondary to a deep vein thrombosis. He has a history of chronic kidney disease and his eGFR is less than 30.
- For this reason dalteparin is contraindicated and unfractionated heparin (infusion) should be used.

Q2
The correct answer is 'E'.

- This question is testing your ability to manage a tachycardia and, in particular, atrial fibrillation.
- The ALS tachycardia algorithm defines management according to the presence of adverse signs (heart failure, myocardial ischaemia, shock and syncope), and whether the QRS complexes are narrow or broad. In this case there are no 'adverse signs' and we do not know when the atrial fibrillation commenced, so cardioversion without prior anti-coagulation is contraindicated.
- Rate control is therefore the preferred option, and oral metoprolol is the correct option.

Q3
The correct answer is 'C'.

- Benzodiazepine medication (including temazepam) is indicated for use as a short-term anxiolytic and hypnotic. Sudden withdrawal of the medication in long-term users is associated with an acute confusion and, rarely, even suicide.
- The correct way to manage these patients is to switch the benzodiazepine drug to diazepam at a recommended conversion rate (BNF) and then taper off gradually.
- The long-term effects of chronic benzodiazepine use include dependency, cognitive impairment (22) and falls.
- Zopiclone has a similar effect to benzodiazepines and so conversion to this is not recommended (23).

Q4
The correct answer is 'E'.

- This child has presented with what seems like acute severe asthma, as indicated by respiratory distress, RR >30 bpm, pulse >125 bpm, hypotension, SpO_2 <92% and not being able to speak in full sentences.

- According to BTS/SIGN Guidelines (24), we should do the following:
  - Give a beta-2 agonist such as salbutamol either as an increasing inhaled dose (up to a maximum of 10 puffs) or as 2.5–5 mg of salbutamol, preferably via an oxygen-driven nebulizer. The latter is the better option in this case as inhaled salbutamol has not been effective prior to admission.
- Following the above, there is also evidence that use of an anti-muscarinic bronchodilator such as ipratropium bromide every 20–30 minutes in the first 2 hours of a severe asthma attack in addition to the beta-2 agonist is safe and efficacious in controlling the symptoms.
- Early corticosteroid doses can help prevent a relapse, and an effect is noticed within 3–4 hours. Where oral doses are not tolerated, an intravenous dose of hydrocortisone (at 4 mg/kg to a maximum of 100 mg every 6 hours) can be utilized.
- In unresponsive or life-threatening cases, the child should be transferred to a high-dependency or intensive care area, and parenteral treatment with salbutamol or aminophylline should be initiated.

Q5
The correct answer is 'D'.

- The most appropriate option is to give an intravenous bolus of 10–20 mL/kg of 0.9% sodium chloride; this can be repeated if needed. Use of glucose 10% is not appropriate unless there are electrolyte issues, the patient has a metabolic disorder or the patient is a neonate.
- Dehydration will need to be considered when calculating the fluid requirements (hence, two-thirds maintenance is not correct in this instance).
- A hypotonic solution of sodium chloride is used in some neonatal units (for pre-term babies and neonates in intensive care areas). It is not used routinely in those with low sodium levels due to risk of further hyponatraemia leading to cerebral oedema and death.
- The full safety advice on 'hypotonic saline' issued in 2012 can be accessed via Ref. (25).

Q6
The correct answer is 'C'.

- Conservative management with pain relief and support is the most appropriate option currently; however, patient consultation will then deem the next step (i.e. medical management, surgical intervention or natural course of events without intervention).
- A second USS can be utilized if it is requested for reassurance purposes.

Q7

The correct answer is 'E'.

- Although options A and C are plausible, they are not the most appropriate in this instance.
- Option B is clearly inappropriate as this patient should have consultant-led care in hospital.
- We should start her on medication to help control her liver condition and resulting pruritus which is clearly a case of obstetric cholestasis.
- Use of a topical emollient will provide short-term relief, whereas using a bile sequestrant such as ursodeoxycholic acid will be more useful in the long term.
- For more information, refer to Ref. (26).

Q8

The correct answer is 'E'.

- This patient is presenting with a tricyclic antidepressant overdose; the purpose of active monitoring is to allow accurate assessment of when treatment is required and whether sodium bicarbonate is required.
- The indications for the infusion of sodium bicarbonate in the context of a tricyclic overdose include:
  - Metabolic – acidosis (pH <7.1)
  - Neurological – seizures or neuroexcitablity
  - Cardiac – broad QRS/arrhythmia
  - Hypotension
- Amiodarone can be used to treat ventricular tachycardia, though in the context of tricyclic overdose the best option is sodium bicarbonate.

COMMUNICATING INFORMATION

Q1
The correct answer is 'C'.

Option A	Folic acid supplementation is doubly important as neural tube defects are more common with anticonvulsants.
Option B	National statistics are important for public health research purposes.
Option C	Specialist advice is required on adjusting medications to minimize risk to unborn foetus as well as the mother and so this is the most important information that must be communicated.
Option D	Sodium valproate is the safest of all the anticonvulsants, but wouldn't be initiated in general practice.
Option E	Most anticonvulsants are teratogenic and the risk to foetus is greater than that to the mother.

Q2
The correct answer is 'B'.

Option A	Eye drops may contain preservatives which can accumulate if a patient wears contact lenses in the daytime and cause toxicity.
Option B	Patients must be counselled about a change in eye colour with prostaglandin drops, especially those patients applying unilaterally.
Option C	Eye drops can have systemic absorption and hence prostaglandin can affect smooth muscle in asthmatics.
Option D	Local small-vessel absorption can trigger headaches.
Option E	Systemic effects include raising the blood pressure; therefore, heightened awareness is required in hypertensives.

Q3
The correct answer is 'A'.

Option A	Topical chloramphenicol is a valid empirical treatment in a child with signs of acute conjunctivitis, even <1. The risk of aplastic anaemia is not thought to be significant anymore.
Option B	Topical fusidic acid is also a valid empirical treatment, usually when a staphylococcal infection is suspected, and the lesser frequency required compared to chloramphenicol makes it arguably more practically viable in a <1 year old.
Option C	Empirical treatment is reasonable in these circumstances unless ophthalmia neonatorum is suspected.
Option D	Nasolacrimal duct obstruction in a young child <1 is possible, but the symptoms of a persistently mucoid discharge in the lacrimal duct are usually a key feature of this from a few weeks of age.
Option E	A vertical transmission of an STI from mother to baby is possible but only in the first few days after birth.

Q4
The correct answer is 'B'.

Option A	According to the Department of Health guidance, which is updated yearly and accessible via Ref. (27), a 12-month-old child should receive the following vaccinations:
Option B	• Hib/MenC vaccine (single booster dose) – inactivated vaccine • Pneumococcal vaccine (single booster dose) – inactivated vaccine • MMR vaccine (first dose) – live vaccine
Option C	Concerns regarding the safety of the MMR vaccine have now been discredited, and there is no causal link between the vaccine and autism.
Option D	It is not necessary to postpone doses in children without any fever or systemic basis to their illness.
Option E	Childhood immunization vaccines should be obtained from local health organizations or from ImmForm (www.immform.dh.gov.uk) and should not be prescribed on an FP10.

When two or more vaccines are to be administered, they should be given at different sites. Where two vaccines are administered in the same limb, they should be given at least 2.5 cm apart. Where two live parenteral vaccines (note – this does not apply to live oral vaccines) cannot be given together, they should be given at least 4 weeks apart unless specified otherwise (28).

Q5
The correct answer is 'A'.

Option A	Alcohol products (this can be medication, mouthwashes etc.) should be avoided while on metronidazole and for 48 hours after the course has completed due to the inherent risk of a 'disulfiram-like reaction' consisting of flushing, headache and tachycardia, among others. Metronidazole carries warning label 4: Do not drink alcohol.
Option B	She should complete her full course (unless advised otherwise by a medical professional) even if she starts to feel better, as the risks of recurrence and resistance are enhanced if she stops the course. Metronidazole carries advisory label 9: Space the doses evenly throughout the day. Keep taking this medicine until the course is finished, unless you are told to stop.
Option C	The tablets should be taken with or after food due to the risk of GI side effects. A small amount of food (e.g. a biscuit, piece of toast etc.) is usually sufficient. Metronidazole carries advisory label 21: Take with or just after food, or a meal.
Option D	Metronidazole tablets can decrease taste acuity or alter sensation of taste and so it will taste unpleasant if crushed or chewed.
Option E	Metronidazole tablets are taken with plenty of water (at least 150 mL; some literature says 240 mL) to prevent irritation of the oesophagus and stomach. Metronidazole carries advisory label 27: Take with a full glass of water.

Q6
The correct answer is 'B'.

Option A	Although it is correct that a rash and loss of libido can be side effects of SSRIs, they are not the most important facts to warn the patient about when initiating these drugs.
Option B	A recent meta-analysis showed that the risk of sudden-onset suicidal thoughts started on SSRIs is not just present in the under 18s, but also significantly raised in 18–24 year olds (MHRA, 2014), and patients need to be counselled on this point at initiation.
Option C	SSRIs do not interact with dietary tyramine to cause a hypertensive crisis; however, the MAOI class of antidepressant does.
Option D	Although it is correct that SSRIs do interact with tricyclic antidepressants to increase the risk of serotonin syndrome, this is not the most important piece of information to warn the patient about.
Option E	SSRIs do cause a loss of libido, but again this tends not to be a side effect that patients report in the early stages of treatment.

CALCULATIONS

Q1

Correct answer

5.5 mL

Working

70×3 = maximum dose = 210 mg
5 mL of 2% lidocaine solution is 100 mg of lidocaine.
Thus, the remaining mass of lidocaine is 110 mg which is 5.5 mL.

Q2

Correct answer

220 mg

Working

First convert all formulations to morphine dosage per 24 hours:
75 micrograms/hour fentanyl patch = 300 mg morphine sulphate/24 hours
15 mg oral morphine every hour = 24 hours $\times$ 15 mg = 360 mg
Total = 660 mg morphine sulphate/24 hours
Diamorphine 10 mg = morphine sulphate 30 mg
Therefore the ratio is 1:3.
660/3 = diamorphine/24 hours = 220 mg

Q3

Correct answer

20 drops

Working

1 drop of alfacalcidol (2 micrograms/mL) contains approximately 100 nanograms/drop.
2 micrograms = 2000 nanograms
2000/100 = 20 drops

Q4

Correct answer

2

Working

Suitable quantities of corticosteroid preparations to be prescribed for specific areas of the body and sufficient for a single daily application in an adult (over a 2-week application period):

Area	Creams and ointments
Scalp OR both hands OR face and neck OR groins and genitalia	15–30 g
Both arms	30–60 g
Both legs OR trunk	100 g

Proportionally smaller amounts are needed in children.

Both hands	15–30 g
Both arms	30–60 g
Trunk	100 g

Total range = (15 to 30 g) + (30 to 60 g) + (100 g) = 145 to 190 g, hence two tubes are needed.

Q5

Correct answer

BSA = 2.53 m²

Working

$$BSA = \sqrt{(160 \times 145)/(3600)}$$
$$= \sqrt{(23200)/(3600)}$$
$$= \sqrt{(232)/(36)}$$

A BNF calculator for BSA is available to healthcare professionals on:
https://www.medicinescomplete.com/mc/bnf/current/
(Scroll to bottom of page to the section titled 'supplementary information', and click on calculators.)

Q6

Correct answer

90 mg

Working

BSA = 1.77 m²
Dose = 50 × 1.77 = 88.5 mg
A good dose to give is 90 mg.
A BNF calculator for BSA is available to healthcare professionals on:
https://www.medicinescomplete.com/mc/bnf/current/
(Scroll to bottom of page to the section titled 'supplementary information', and click on calculators.)

Q7

Correct answer

7.2 mL

Working

Trimethoprim dosing for this child is 4 mg/kg (max. 200 mg) every 12 hours.
Child weight can be estimated by the formula: (age + 4) × 2.
Therefore the child weighs (5 + 4) × 2 = 18 kg.
Child needs 18 × 4 = 72 mg BD.
Trimethoprim suspension preparation is 50 mg/5 mL (≡10 mg in 1 mL).
Hence 72 mg will be in 7.2 mL.

- Most localities have developed antimicrobial guidelines for primary care. An example is the SW London Guidelines, adapted from the template Public Health England document (29). This gives excellent guidance on first-line, second-line and third-line antimicrobials for various common infections encountered in the community, and they vary due to differences in local resistances. For UTI in this age group it also advises when and when not to prescribe antibiotics empirically by describing the negative predictive value (NPV) of the dipstick result.

- The NICE guidelines for UTI in children aged over 3 years (30) have recently changed. For a non-recurrent UTI, referral for advanced imaging to paediatrics is no longer recommended. Imaging is only required for a recurrent UTI, unless it is an atypical (non-*E. coli*) infection, in which case an urgent USS is the imaging of choice.

Q8

Correct answer

525–700 micrograms (dose range)

Working

Dose range = 150–200 micrograms/kg
3.5 × 150 = 525 micrograms
3.5 × 200 = 700 micrograms

ADVERSE DRUG REACTIONS

Q1

The correct answer is 'B'.

- Clindamycin is frequently associated with diarrhoea and antibiotic-associated colitis, which necessitate treatment cessation.
- Gentamicin (an aminoglycoside anti-infective agent) can cause all of the other listed side effects and should be avoided in those with renal failure. Ototoxicity with aminoglycosides is irreversible.

Q2

The correct answer is 'A'.

- The most likely side effects of hormone replacement therapy with Evorel® Conti are nausea, vomiting, abdominal cramps, breast tenderness, pre-menstrual-like syndrome, sodium and fluid retention, jaundice, glucose intolerance and an altered lipid profile.
- Headache, dizziness and leg cramp (attempt to rule out DVT) can also occur.
- Patches may lead to contact sensitization and headache on vigorous exercise.
- Long-term use can lead to an increased risk of options B to E.

Q3

The correct answer is 'E'.

- Epleronone is an aldosterone antagonist, similar in function to spironolactone. It is used in patients with a reduced left ventricular ejection fraction (e.g. less than 40%) after myocardial infarction. It is most likely to cause hyperkalaemia through its potassium-sparing action on the kidney.
- Trimethoprim can also cause hyperkalaemia even if the patient has only taken the antibiotic for 2 days.
- Candesartan is an angiotensin receptor blocker (ARB) and can also cause hyperkalaemia.
- Furosemide causes potassium wasting, so it would have the opposite effect.

Q4

The correct answer is 'C'.

- This woman's rash has the typical description of psoriasis.
- This type of rash can be caused by lithium as well as some other drug groups (e.g. beta-blockers and, less commonly, ACEIs).
- Most drug reaction rashes occur within a few days of starting the medication; however, in the case of a psoriatic rash, it can take up to months.

Q5

The correct answer is 'B'.

- Clozapine is one of the second-generation antipsychotics.
- There are three major precautions that have to be considered for any patient on one of these medications, relating to the blood, the heart and the bowels.
- The medication is usually started in secondary care, so a GP needs to be aware of these side effects to monitor its use adequately.
- The blood can be affected by agranulocytosis, the heart can develop cardiomyositis and the bowels can rarely develop paralytic ileus but more commonly constipation.
- A good way to screen for the cardiac complications is checking for tachycardia.

Q6

The correct answer is 'E'.

- This woman has developed symptoms of serotonin syndrome due to the interaction between citalopram and tramadol.
- Tramadol has a dual action of pain relief – it is an opioid analgesic but also works as a serotonin and noradrenaline reuptake inhibitor.
- The increased risk of death, especially in overdose, with tramadol was highlighted recently, and therefore it became upgraded to a Class C drug by the Royal Pharmaceutical Society in 2014.
- As a result of this, restrictions apply that it should not be given for longer than 28 days per prescription, it should not be put onto a repeat prescription and it cannot be prescribed electronically (EPS).

Q7

The correct answer is 'E'.

- Toxic epidermal necrolysis is a blistering condition of the skin leading to loss of skin barrier function.
- The treatment of the condition are largely supportive, including:
  - Barrier nursing to limit infection
  - Warming measures to promote skin growth
  - Fluid support to replace cutaneous losses
  - Analgesia
  - Dressing of wounds
- Steroids and immunosuppressants are not routinely indicated in the treatment of the disease, and neither is surgical de-roofing of blisters.

Q8

The correct answer is 'A'.

- Metoclopramide is known to cause extrapyramidal side effects (as described in the scenario) and is the most likely culprit in children and young adults aged 15–19 years.
- Reactions tend to occur shortly after treatment initiation, but subside within 24 hours of drug withdrawal. For more on the safety information associated with this drug, see Ref. (31).
- The treatment for this condition includes anticholinergic therapies (benztropine) and anti-histamines. Promethazine is occasionally used.
- The MHRA and CHM advise that metoclopramide should be used in the short term only (for up to 5 days).
- Cyclizine can in rare cases also cause extrapyramidal side effects and this may need to be considered as an alternative culprit (although not the most likely one).

DRUG MONITORING

Q1
The correct answer is 'C'.

- In a patient stating that they have 'erratic blood sugars', it is important to establish whether hypoglycaemia has occurred.
- In the management of diabetes, *hypo*glycaemia will cause serious morbidity or even mortality more quickly than *hyper*glycaemia.
- The other options are important to monitor in terms of diabetic control, but the option that is most concerned with immediate danger is C.

Q2
The correct answer is 'D'.

- The Disease Activity Score 28 is a conjugate measure used in rheumatoid arthritis.
- It includes a clinical examination of 28 joints and of serum measures of inflammation (including CRP or erythrocyte sedimentation rate), and it is recommended by Ref. (32).

Q3
The correct answer is 'E'.

- Tenofovir is a nucleotide analogue reverse transcriptase inhibitor. It is associated with renal impairment due to damage sustained to the proximal tubule which can progress to Fanconi syndrome. For this reason the British HIV Association (BHIVA) recommends 3–6 monthly monitoring of urinalysis for evidence of tubular damage (protein or blood in the urine).

Q4
The correct answer is 'E'.

- Statins have two side effects that need to be monitored for:
  - Effects on the liver
  - Skeletal muscle effects (rhabdomyolysis)
- Should the ALT/AST levels rise to >3 times the normal, then the statin should be stopped. It is otherwise not considered to be significant (17).
- Should the patient develop muscle pains, then a CK rise will help decide if the statin is the cause. Remember that a higher CK can be normal in Afro-Caribbeans.
- CK need not be checked in asymptomatic patients and a rise of >5 times the baseline is considered a significant rise.

Q5

The correct answer is 'A'.

- Theophylline is a methyl-xanthine that is used in severe asthma attacks.
- The therapeutic range is narrow (10–20 mmol/L), and beyond this range toxicity and adverse effects are more likely.
- This patient is elderly and has heart failure and possible liver impairment; therefore, the risk of toxicity is higher.
- Cardiac parameters (i.e. pulse, heart rate and blood pressure) will give earliest signs of adverse effects.

Q6

The correct answer is 'E'.

- Quetiapine is a second-generation (or atypical) antipsychotic. It works more selectively as a dopamine antagonist in comparison to the first-generation antipsychotics, as well as a 5HT and histamine receptor antagonist. Consequently it can have an impact on BMI and has an increased risk of diabetes.
- It can also cause ECG abnormalities and affect the lipid profile, hence the need for an annual CVD risk assessment. It is known that a patient with severe mental health illness has a 15–20 year shorter life expectancy than an age-matched patient not on the severe mental health disease register.
- It can also cause leucopenia although not as dramatically as clozapine.
- For this reason GPs are asked to perform the above monitoring prior to a mental health review.

Q7

The correct answer is 'D'.

- Assessment of acidosis occurs once serum glucose and ketones have been determined. Diabetic ketoacidosis is characterized by a venous pH of less than 7.3 or a bicarbonate level of <15 mmol/L in addition to the presence of blood (or urinary) ketones.
- Hyperglycaemia can lead to urinary calcium loss; however, this will not always manifest as a drop in serum calcium due to calcium in other parts of the body (e.g. bones).
- Potassium levels need to be checked as they drop in cases of diabetic ketoacidosis (DKA) and also because if there is any acidosis that is being corrected, this will also lead to further drops. For this reason, potassium-based infusions are used in cases of DKA unless levels are high or the patient is anuric. A cardiac monitor can be used in patients with DKA to assess for signs of hyper- or hypo-kalaemia.
- Blood glucose (and urinary ketone testing) is needed initially. If blood glucose is ≥11 mmol/L and ketone levels are >0.6 mmol/L, the test is positive for diabetic ketoacidosis.
- A blood culture is not needed unless there are any clinical signs of either sepsis or an infection.

The correct answer is 'A'.

- The beneficial effect of this treatment will be apparent from a reduction in the erythrocyte sedimentation rate which is a marker of inflammation. Sometimes plasma viscosity (PV), which is purported to be a more superior test, is monitored.
- The other monitoring options are necessary to ensure safe prescribing and to notice any adverse effects. For example, renal and liver impairment will necessitate a dose reduction or withholding of treatment as would a rise in the white cell count.
- Other side effects of treatment such as stomatitis, nausea, vomiting, headaches and mild hair loss can be managed with a once-daily dose of folic acid taken on 3–6 days of the week (but not on the day of methotrexate dosing). Pulmonary toxicity can occur; symptoms include a persistent dry unproductive cough and dyspnoea.
- Methotrexate is given ONCE WEEKLY and can be fatal in overdose (e.g. if given once daily).
- Patients should carry their 'purple book' with them at all times when they go to see their doctor, pharmacist or nurse.
- Other drugs that require patients to carry an 'alert card' or 'record book' include:

Drug/class of drug	Card/book needed
Warfarin	Yellow 'alert card' and 'oral anti-coagulation therapy' booklet
Lithium	Lithium 'alert card' and 'record book'
Corticosteroids	Blue 'steroid card'
Apixaban, dabigatran and rivaroxaban	Patient 'alert card'
Insulin	Insulin passport
Oxygen	Oxygen 'alert card'

DATA INTERPRETATION

Q1

The correct answer is 'D'.

- The gram-negative diplococci with the leukocyte-heavy urine dip point towards *Neisseria gonorrhoea* infection.
- The recommended treatment is therefore an intramuscular injection of cefalexin followed by a course of oral azithromycin.

Q2

The correct answer is 'B'.

- The importance in this case is to adequately cover the possible causative organisms.
- The ultrasound and blood results point towards a diagnosis of biliary sepsis with likely organisms being gram-negatives but definitely requiring anaerobic cover with metronidazole.
- This patient is penicillin allergic, meaning that cephalosporins (such as ceftriaxone) should also be avoided due to a degree of crossover.
- Ciprofloxacin has the same bioavailability orally as intravenously and is associated with injection site reactions, so it is best given via an oral route.

Q3

The correct answer is 'C'.

- The patient described has a hypochloraemic, hypokalaemic alkalosis secondary to vomiting. This is due to the loss of potassium chloride (an acid) from the stomach due to vomiting and likely potassium loss due to diarrhoea.
- Other causes of hypochloraemic, hypokalaemic alkalosis include diuretics, Barter's syndrome and Gittleman's syndrome.
- The important elements to managing this condition are:
  - Replace potassium – particularly as she has ECG evidence of hypokalaemia.
  - Replace fluid losses – she has clinical findings of dehydration (low JVP, dry mucosae, raised urea and raised lactate).
  - The correct management is therefore to give lots of fluid (1 L rather than 500 mL), with potassium and chloride (contained in normal saline and not in 5% dextrose). Hartmann's contains approximately 5 mmol potassium, far less than would be delivered in a bag containing 40 mmol. This option is therefore incorrect.

Q4

The correct answer is 'D'.

- In this case the patient is over-oxygenated, with an inappropriately low respiratory rate for the high level of carbon dioxide.

- The raised bicarbonate suggests a chronic metabolic compensation for chronically raised carbon dioxide, so it is likely that the patient has lost the hypercapnoeic element of respiratory drive.
- He does not have type II respiratory failure and so does not require non-invasive ventilation.
- The delivery of oxygen needs to be reduced and carefully titrated.
- A Venturi mask enables an exact FiO_2 of oxygen to be delivered, and a 28% mask would be a reduction from 5 L/min.

Q5
The correct answer is 'C'.

- This woman has developed a persistently elevated BP of >140/90. For this reason she has to stop taking it, although not immediately. The BP cut-off for immediate withdrawal is >160/95.
- She also has other risk factors for arterial disease which, due to the fact that there are more than one of them, necessitate avoiding the COCP. These include in her case her age and her obesity.
- If she was to only have had a persistently raised BP and none of the other factors, she could have continued to use the COCP with monitoring for the immediate cut-off level.
- If the BMI were >35, then that in itself would have necessitated avoidance.
- The POP is permitted as a substitute as it is the oestrogenic component that is causing the risk.
- Women should be advised to report worsening of headaches when on the COCP due to the question of migraine.

Q6
The correct answer is 'D'.

- This child has taken a paracetamol overdose which at 7 hours post ingestion shows a paracetamol concentration level above the cut-off for the antidote of N-acetylcysteine; therefore, it should be commenced.
- Activated charcoal and gastric lavage should only be commenced if the overdose has been taken less than 1 hour before presentation.
- If presenting 8–24 hours post ingestion, then N-acetylcysteine should be commenced without awaiting the levels but stopped if below the cut-off when results are obtained.
- Once N-acetylcysteine has been commenced, it can be expected to be continued for at least 21 hours, except in the circumstances mentioned above.
- Serious signs of a known paracetamol overdose include hypotension, encephalopathy and hepatoxicity.

References

1. Campagna JD, Bond MC, Schabelman E, Hayes BD. The use of cephalosporins in penicillin-allergic patients: A literature review. *J Emerg Med*. 2012; 42(5): 612–20.
2. Baker E, Roberts AP, Wilde K, Walton H, Suri S, Rull G, et al. Development of a core drug list towards improving prescribing education and reducing errors in the UK. *Br J Clin Pharmacol*. 2011; 71(2): 190–8.
3. *Domperidone: Risks of cardiac side effects*. Drug Safety Update – GOV.UK. https://www.gov.uk/drug-safety-update/domperidone-risks-of-cardiac-side-effects
4. *Gastro-oesophageal reflux disease: Recognition, diagnosis and management in children and young people | reflux-in-babies | Information for the public | NICE*. NICE. https://www.nice.org.uk/guidance/ng1/ifp/chapter/reflux-in-babies
5. *Hypertension in pregnancy | Guidance and guidelines | NICE*. NICE. https://www.nice.org.uk/guidance/cg107
6. *Antenatal care | Guidance and guidelines | NICE*. NICE. https://www.nice.org.uk/guidance/cg62
7. *Nausea/vomiting in pregnancy* – NICE CKS. http://cks.nice.org.uk/nauseavomiting-in-pregnancy
8. Hunder GG, Bloch DA, Michel BA, Stevens MB, Arend WP, Calabrese LH, et al. The American College of Rheumatology 1990 criteria for the classification of giant cell arteritis. *Arthritis Rheum*. 1990; 33(8): 1122–8.
9. *Citalopram and escitalopram: QT interval prolongation*. Drug Safety Update – GOV.UK. https://www.gov.uk/drug-safety-update/citalopram-and-escitalopram-qt-interval-prolongation
10. *Pelvic inflammatory disease* – NICE CKS. http://cks.nice.org.uk/pelvic-inflammatory- disease
11. Medicines and Healthcare products Regulatory Agency (MHRA). *Combined oral contraceptives (the pill): When to start taking the pill, and missed pill advice*. London: Medicines and Healthcare products Regulatory Agency (MHRA). http://www.mhra.gov.uk/safety-public-assessment-reports/CON120481
12. Mythen MG, Swart M, Acheson N, Crawford R, Jones K, Kuper M, et al. Perioperative fluid management: Consensus statement from the enhanced recovery partnership. *Perioper Med (London, England)*. 2012; 1: 2.
13. De Ruiter A, Taylor GP, Clayden P, Dhar J, Gandhi K, Gilleece Y, et al. British HIV Association guidelines for the management of HIV infection in pregnant women 2012 (2014 interim review). *HIV Med*. 2014; 15(Suppl 4): 1–77.
14. *Simvastatin: Updated advice on drug interactions*. Drug Safety Update – GOV.UK. https://www.gov.uk/drug-safety-update/simvastatin-updated-advice-on-drug-interactions
15. *Hydroxychloroquine and ocular toxicity recommendations on screening*. The Royal College of Ophthalmologists. https://www.rcophth.ac.uk/wp-content/uploads/2014/12/2009-SCI-010-Ocular-Toxicity.pdf
16. *Bipolar disorder: The management of bipolar disorder in adults, children and adolescents, in primary and secondary care | important-information-about-this-guidance | Guidance and guidelines | NICE*. NICE. https://www.nice.org.uk/guidance/cg38
17. *Lipid modification: Cardiovascular risk assessment and the modification of blood lipids for the primary and secondary prevention of cardiovascular disease | Guidance and guidelines | NICE*. NICE. https://www.nice.org.uk/guidance/cg181

18. *Pyelonephritis – Acute – NICE CKS.* http://cks.nice.org.uk/pyelonephritis-acute#! scenario/

19. *Impetigo – NICE CKS.* http://cks.nice.org.uk/impetigo#!topicsummary

20. *Constipation – NICE CKS.* http://cks.nice.org.uk/constipation

21. *Unstable angina and NSTEMI.* NICE. https://www.nice.org.uk/guidance/cg94

22. Billioti de Gage S, Moride Y, Ducruet T, Kurth T, Verdoux H, Tournier M, et al. Benzodiazepine use and risk of Alzheimer's disease: Case-control study. *BMJ.* 2014; 349: g5205.

23. *Guidance on the use of zaleplon, zolpidem and zopiclone for the short-term management of insomnia | Guidance and guidelines | NICE.* NICE. https://www.nice.org.uk/guidance/ta77

24. British Thoracic Society, Scottish Intercollegiate Guidelines Network. British guideline on the management of asthma. *Thorax.* 2003; 58(Suppl 1): i1–94.

25. *Intravenous 0.18% saline/4% glucose solution ("hypotonic saline") in children: Reports of fatal hyponatraemia.* Drug Safety Update – GOV.UK. https://www.gov.uk/drug-safety-update/intravenous-0-18-saline-4-glucose-solution-hypotonic-saline-in-children-reports-of-fatal-hyponatraemia

26. *Obstetric cholestasis (green-top guideline no. 43).* https://www.rcog.org.uk/en/guidelines-research-services/guidelines/gtg43/

27. *The complete routine immunisation schedule – Publications – GOV.UK.* https://www.gov.uk/government/publications/the-complete-routine-immunisation-schedule

28. Revised recommendations for the administration of more than one live vaccine. Public Health England. https://www.gov.uk/government/uploads/system/uploads/attachment_data/file/422798/PHE_recommendations_for_administering_more_than_one_live_vaccine_April_2015FINAL_.pdf

29. *Managing common infections: Guidance for primary care.* Public Health England. https://www.gov.uk/government/publications/managing-common-infections-guidance-for-primary-care

30. *Urinary tract infection in children | Guidance and guidelines | NICE.* NICE. https://www.nice.org.uk/guidance/cg54

31. *Metoclopramide: Risk of neurological adverse effects.* Drug Safety Update – GOV.UK. https://www.gov.uk/drug-safety-update/metoclopramide-risk-of-neurological-adverse-effects

32. Anderson J, Caplan L, Yazdany J, Robbins ML, Neogi T, Michaud K, et al. Rheumatoid arthritis disease activity measures: American College of Rheumatology recommendations for use in clinical practice. *Arthritis Care Res (Hoboken).* 2012; 64(5): 640–7.

Index